Handbook of Hospice Policies and Procedures

Marilyn D. Harris, RN, MSN, CNAA, FAAN
Executive Director
Abington Memorial Hospital Home Care
Willow Grove, Pennsylvania

Elissa Della Monica, RN, MSN, CNA
Director of Professional Services
Abington Memorial Hospital Home Care
Willow Grove, Pennsylvania

Pamela Boyd, RN, MSN, RNH
Hospice Supervisor
Abington Memorial Hospital Home Care
Willow Grove, Pennsylvania

AN ASPEN PUBLICATION®
Aspen Publishers, Inc.
Gaithersburg, Maryland
1999

This publication is designed to provide accurate and authoritative information in regard to the Subject Matter covered. It is sold with the understanding that the publisher is not engaged in rendering legal, accounting, or other professional service. If legal advice or other expert assistance is required, the service of a competent professional person should be sought. (From a Declaration of Principles jointly adopted by a Committee of the American Bar Association and a Committee of Publishers and Associations.)

Library of Congress Cataloging-in-Publication Data

Harris, Marilyn D.
Handbook of hospice policies and procedures / Marilyn D. Harris, Elissa Della Monica, Pamela Boyd.
p. cm.
Includes bibliographical references and index.
ISBN 0-8342-1329-X
1. Hospice care—Handbooks, manuals, etc. 2. Hospices (Terminal care)—Handbooks, manuals, etc.
I. Della Monica, Elissa. II. Boyd, Pamela. III. Title.
H726.8.H366 1999
362.1'756—dc21
99-13888
CIP

Copyright © 1999 by Aspen Publishers, Inc.
All rights reserved.

Aspen Publishers, Inc., grants permission for photocopying for limited personal or internal use. This consent does not extend to other kinds of copying, such as copying for general distribution, for advertising or promotional purposes, for creating new collective works, or for resale. For information, address Aspen Publishers, Inc., Permissions Department, 200 Orchard Ridge Drive, Suite 200, Gaithersburg, Maryland 20878.

All forms, policies, and procedures in this publication are courtesy of Abington Memorial Hospital, Willow Grove, Pennsylvania. Copyright © 1998. All rights reserved.

Orders: (800) 638-8437
Customer Service: (800) 234-1660

About Aspen Publishers • For more than 35 years, Aspen has been a leading professional publisher in a variety of disciplines. Aspen's vast information resources are available in both print and electronic formats. We are committed to providing the highest quality information available in the most appropriate format for our customers. Visit Aspen's Internet site for more information resources, directories, articles, and a searchable version of Aspen's full catalog, including the most recent publications: **http://www.aspenpublishers.com**
Aspen Publishers, Inc. • The hallmark of quality in publishing
Member of the worldwide Wolters Kluwer group.

Editorial Services: Joan Sesma
Library of Congress Catalog Card Number: 99-13888
ISBN: 0-8342-1329-X

Printed in the United States of America

1 2 3 4 5

TABLE OF CONTENTS

Acknowledgments v

Introduction vii

How To Use This Handbook xi

Bibliography xiii

Acronyms and Abbreviations xv

PART I—Policies and Procedures 1

PART II—Forms 141

PART III—List of Medicare Conditions of Participation Cross-References ... 199

Appendix A—Federal Register Material 201

Index 263

ACKNOWLEDGMENTS

The administrative and supervisory staff of the Abington Memorial Hospital Home Care (AMHHC) Hospice Program acknowledge the support of The Abington Memorial Hospital administration, the AMHHC Professional Advisory Committee, and the Hospice Interdisciplinary Team in the preparation, review, and approval of policies and procedures.

The editors also thank all members of the Hospice team for their commitment to provide high-quality care and support to the hundreds of individuals and their families who choose the Abington Memorial Hospital Home Care Hospice Program each year.

INTRODUCTION

INTRODUCTION

A current policy manual is essential for the administration and service delivery of home health/hospice care. *Webster's Ninth New Collegiate Dictionary*[1] defines a policy as "providence or wisdom in the management of affairs; a definite course or method of action selected from among alternatives in light of given conditions to guide and determined present and future decisions; a high-level overall plan embracing the general goals and acceptable procedures."

Rowland and Rowland[2] advised that there are three general areas of nursing that require policy formulation: areas in which confusion about the focus of responsibility might result in neglect or malperformance of an act necessary to a patient's welfare, areas pertaining to the protection of patient's and family's rights, and areas involving matters of personnel management and welfare.

Barnum and Kerfoot[3] state that a policy is a guideline that has been formalized by administrative authority and directs action to some purpose. Policies should be revised periodically for efficiency, safety, and effectiveness. There are three major components in a policy system: a purpose, a policy role, and an action directive or procedure. A procedure details the means to be used to achieve the ends specified in the purpose and further delineated in the policy.

Perrow[4] states that policy rules are necessary in complex organizations due to such things as variability in personnel, clients, and environment. These policies delineate an area of freedom where staff members know when they can make decisions. The absence of written policy leaves staff in a position where any decision they make may infringe upon an unstated policy and produce a reprimand.

Before any service is provided, an approved policy must be in place. This policy gives direction to staff as to what services will be provided under what conditions. It also should state what is not provided and the rationale, if appropriate. Care must be taken to make a policy specific while allowing for flexibility to meet specific situations that may arise.

POLICY DEVELOPMENT

The development of a policy can take several forms. First, staff at all levels may identify a need to provide a specific service. This could be done through systematic logging of requests for service that is not already available through the agency. Information can be gathered from staff about the volume of requests for the new service and also about the rationale. A review of the literature or contact with other agencies that provide the service and their success or failure rate with this service is also beneficial. If staff initiate the request for a policy, it can be anticipated that some preliminary homework has been done to substantiate the request.

Second, physicians, or other referral sources, may request that personnel perform a specific service. If the request is initiated from an outside source, staff who are knowledgeable in the specific procedure under discussion should be involved in the development of the policy.

Third, policies can be developed as a result of the internal quality assessment/performance improvement (QA/PI) program. Specific areas of concern may be identified through the quarterly record or utilization review process that could benefit from a new or revised policy.

Multiple levels of home health/hospice personnel should be involved in the revisions or deletions of policies from an agency's manual as well as the development of new ones.

The staff from both home health agencies and hospice programs care for individuals with a terminal illness. Medicare regulations state that the certified hospice interdisciplinary group (IDG) is responsible for development of policies and procedures for the day-to-day provision of hospice care and services.

One important aspect of the development of sound policies is to include professionals and lay personnel with a wide array of expertise in multiple areas of current or projected services. This expertise should be available at the staff, contract, committee, and board levels. All individuals, whether on a paid or volunteer basis, are interested in the association they serve and the patients who benefit from these services.

REVIEW AND APPROVAL PROCESS

Policies can be reviewed on an ongoing basis so that all are reviewed annually. Existing clinical service policies should be reviewed by representatives from that discipline to ensure that they are in keeping with current professional standards. Policies such as admission, discharge, and personnel qualifications should be reviewed by appropriate committees from the governing body as well as by administrative staff. Still other policies may need to be reviewed by legal counsel. At other times, an agency administrator may need or want to seek expert advice from an outside consultant such as an insurance carrier for related policies.

The approval process can take several directions depending on the type of agency and policy. Ultimately, the governing body/individual is responsible for approval. This body may not have the expertise to develop or revise specific policies (i.e., use of infusion pumps). For Medicare-certified home health agencies, the Conditions of Participation (COP 486.16)[5] require that an agency have a group of professional personnel, many times referred to as a professional advisory committee (PAC). The PAC is to establish and review the agency's policies related to scope of services, admission and discharge criteria, clinical records, and other related issues. The PAC should meet frequently enough to fulfill its responsibilities.

The Medicare program Conditions of Participation Hospice Care Final Rules (Section 418.68)[6] states that the hospice must designate an IDG or groups that include at least the following individuals who are employees of the hospice: a doctor of medicine or osteopathy, a registered nurse, a social worker, and a pastoral or other counselor. The IDG is responsible for (1) participation in the establishment of the plan of care, (2) provision or supervision of hospice care and services, (3) periodic review and updating of the plan of care for each individual receiving hospice care, and (4) establishment of policies governing the day-to-day provision of hospice care and services. If a hospice has more than one IDG, it must designate in advance the group it chooses to execute the functions described above.

To make the best use of meeting time and to facilitate approval, copies of the proposed policies or changes to existing policies should be mailed to the committee with the agenda prior to the meeting. If there is an age- or disease-specific policy, it is helpful to have a knowledgeable staff person discuss the change and the rationale with the professional on the committee who has expertise in this area. With this prior knowledge, this individual's support can be beneficial at the time of the stated meeting.

For existing policies that are specific to a discipline or department, such as therapy or nursing, representatives from those disciplines should review these. Their comments and suggestions are then shared with the PAC and/or IDG and board for approval. The appropriate board committees should review other policies, such as budget preparation or personnel. Legal counsel should review others, independently or in cooperation with other committees. At other times, an agency may need or want to seek expert advice from an outside consultant, such as an insurance carrier for related policies.

After review by the appropriate committee, recommendations are brought to the governing body via minutes and discussion by the administrative staff for final approval. Board committees and the governing body should meet on a scheduled basis that provides for timely approval of new or revised policies. The hospice IDG and home health PAC review and approve all policies and procedures that govern the operation and service on an annual basis.

CONCLUSION

Sound policies and procedures are important for several reasons, including risk management and to meet state and federal regulations and accreditation, agency, and professional standards. Once these policies are in place they must be communicated and made available to all levels of personnel in the agency so that compliance is ensured.

Although the final approval of policies is the responsibility of the governing body/individual, the recommendation for the development of new policies and revisions to existing policies is a team effort. All levels of personnel within a home health agency and hospice must share ideas that will keep the agency current and competitive with other home care providers.

Whether it is the home health agency's PAC or the hospice IDG that approves service policies and procedures, these approved policies must be communicated to all agency personnel and followed by those to whom they apply. An agency's policy and procedures manual does not belong on the library shelf. It should be readily available to all staff and referred to on a frequent basis by all personnel.

REFERENCES

1. *Webster's Ninth New Collegiate Dictionary* (Springfield, MA: G&C Merriam Co., 1984).
2. S. Rowland and B. Rowland. *Nursing Administration Handbook*, 3d ed. (Gaithersburg, MD: Aspen Publishers, Inc., 1992), 26.
3. B. Barnum and K. Kerfoot, *The Nurse as Executive*, 4th ed. (Gaithersburg, MD: Aspen Publishers, Inc., 1995), 131.
4. C. Perrow, *Complex Organizations* (New York: Random House, 1979), 24.
5. Department of Health and Human Services, Health Care Financing Administration, "Part II. Medicare Program. Home Health Agencies: Conditions of Participation and Reduction in Recordkeeping Requirement: Interim Final Rules," *Federal Register* 54, no. 155 (August 14, 1989): 33354–33373. (42 CFR Part 484. Washington, DC: Government Printing Office).
6. Department of Health and Human Services, Health Care Financing Administration, "Medicare Program: Hospice Care: Final Rule," *Federal Register* 48, no. 243 (December 16, 1983): 56008–56036. (Part VII.) (See Appendix A.)

How To Use This Handbook

The *Handbook of Hospice Policies and Procedures* includes policies, procedures, and forms that address the Medicare Conditions of Participation (COPs), Part 418—Hospice Care.

Subpart B—Eligibility, Election and Duration of Benefits
Subpart C— Conditions of Participation, General Provisions and Administration
Subpart D—Conditions of Participation: Core Services
Subpart E—Conditions of Participation. Other Services

Sample policies, procedures, and forms are from the Abington Memorial Hospital Home Care (AMHHC) Hospice Program, which is Medicare certified and also contracts with health maintenance organizations (HMOs) and indemnity plans to provide hospice care to their subscribers. The AMHHC and hospice programs are accredited with commendation by the Joint Commission on Accreditation of Healthcare Organizations (Joint Commission). The *Handbook of Hospice Policies and Procedures* meets the certification and accreditation standards.

The tables of contents list policies and procedures (Part I) and forms (Part II) in alphabetical order in the *Handbook of Hospice Policies and Procedures* for easy reference. The Hospice Medicare Conditions of Participation are included at the end of each policy or form, when applicable. The tables of contents cross-reference the Medicare Conditions of Participation with the policy and form numbers in this book. In addition, cross-references are included in the tables of contents when the wording of a policy differs from the COP title.

The handbook includes administrative, discipline-specific, and clinical/patient care policies, procedures, and forms. The administrative policies address the organization's philosophy, compliance plan, functions, supervision, patient's rights, staff development, and quality assessment/performance improvement. The discipline-specific policies include the core services and other services that are available through the program. Clinical/patient care policies relate to intake, admission, coordination of care, 24-hour service, physician's orders, and emergency services.

BIBLIOGRAPHY

Balanced Budget Act of 1997. Conference Report to accompany H.R. 2015, U.S. House of Representatives, Report 105-217, July 30, 1997.

Department of Health and Human Services, Health Care Financing Administration, "Medicare Program: Hospice Care," *Federal Register* Vol. 48, No. 243 (December 16, 1983): 56026–56036. (42 CFR Parts 400, 405, 408, 418, 420, 421, 489) Part VII.; Final Rule. (See Appendix A.)

Department of Health and Human Services, Health Care Financing Administration, "Medicare Program: Hospice Care and Prospective Payment for Medicare Inpatient Hospital Services; Correction; Final Rule. Medicare Program; Schedule of Target Rate Percentages for Limits on the Rate of Hospital Cost Increases and Updating Factors for Transition Prospective Payment Rates (Second Quarter FY 84); Correction; Notice," *Federal Register* Vol. 49, No. 107 (June 1, 1984): 23010–23014. (Part VII. 42 CFR Parts 400, 405, 409, 418, 420, 421, 489.) (See Appendix A.)

Department of Health and Human Services, Health Care Financing Administration, "Medicare Program: Hospice Care Services; Nursing," *Federal Register* Vol. 52, No. 47 (March 11, 1987): 7412–7416. (42 CFR Part 418.) (See Appendix A.)

Department of Health and Human Services, Health Care Financing Administration," Medicare Program: Hospice Care Amendments: Medicare," *Federal Register* Vol. 55, No. 238: (December 11, 1990): 50831–50835. (42 CFR Part 418.) (See Appendix A.)

Department of Health and Human Services, Office of Inspector General (OIG), "OIG's Compliance Program Guidance for Home Health Agencies," August 4, 1998: 1–62.

Eli Research, *Home Care Compliance Alert* 2, No. 9 (September 1998) 105–116. Author.

Memorandum from Director, Office of Chronic Care and Insurance Policy, Bureau of Policy Development; Deputy Director for Survey and Certification, Health Standard and Quality Bureau. Subject: Medicare hospice conditions of participation. To All Regional Administrators (June 27, 1997): 1–7.

Acronyms and Abbreviations

Abington Memorial Hospital	AMH
Abington Memorial Hospital Home Care	AMHHC
Activities of Daily Living	ADLs
Animal-Assisted Therapy	AAT
Bedside Commode	BSC
Bureau of Policy Development	BPD
Cardiopulmonary resuscitation	CPR
Centers for Disease Control and Prevention	CDC
Clinical nurse specialist	CNS
Conditions of Participation	COP
Cytomegalovirus	CMV
Department of Environmental Resources	DER
Do not resuscitate	DNR
Durable medical equipment	DME
Emergency room	ER
Food and Drug Administration	FDA
Health Maintenance Organization	HMO
Home Health Standards and Quality Bureau	HSQB
Home health aide	HHA
Homemaker/home health aide	HM/HHA
Human immunodeficiency virus	HIV
Hepatitis B	HBV
Intramuscular	IM
Interdisciplinary group	IDG
Intravenous	IV
Joint Commission on Accreditation of Healthcare Organizations	Joint Commission
Leave of absence	LOA
Licensed Practical Nurse	LPN
Master file input	MFI
Medical assistance	MA
Medical doctor	MD

Medical social worker	MSW
Medicare elect	ME
Nursing	Nsg
Occupational therapy	OT
Omnibus Budget Reconciliation Act	OBRA
Patient master update	PMU
Personal care facility	PCF
Physical therapy	PT
Plan of care	POC
Plan of treatment	POT
Professional advisory committee	PAC
Quality assessment and improvement	QAI
Quality assessment/performance improvement	QA/PI
Skilled nursing facility	SNF
Speech therapy	ST
Telecommunication for the deaf	TTY
Urinary tract infection	UTI
Vital Sign	VS

PART I

Policies and Procedures

Table of Contents

Policy Name	Policy Number	COP
Abington Memorial Hospital Compliance Program	1:01	418.52
Access to Terminal Care Funds	1:02	
Addendum to Clinical Records (also see Levels of Care, 1:40)	1:03	418.74, 418.98
Addressing Ethical Issues	1:04	
Admission Criteria	1:05	418.62
Advance Directives	1:06	418.62
AIDS	1:07	418.14
Bereavement Program	1:08	418.88(a)
Bylaws	1:09	418.52
Clinical Records	1:10	418.74
Communication through Language Interpreters	1:11	418.62
Communication with Visually or Hearing Impaired Patients	1:12	418.62
Competency Evaluation Program	1:13	418.52, 418.56
Conflict of Interest	1:14	418.52
Core Services	1:15	418.80
Death Pronouncement by Registered Nurses	1:16	418.82
Discharge	1:17	418.60
Disposal of Controlled Drugs	1:18	418.96(b)
Disposal of Used Syringes	1:19	418.96
Do Not Resuscitate	1:20	418.62
Eligibility Requirements for Medicare Hospice Benefit	1:21	418.20, 418.24, 418.28
Emergency Phone Numbers	1:22	418.50
Emergency Preparedness Plan	1:23	418.52
Exposure Control Plan	1:24	418.50, 418.66
Governing Body	1:25	418.52

Policy Name	Policy Number	COP
Home Care Services	1:26	418.90, 418.96
Home Health Aide/Homemaker Services	1:27	418.94
Home Health Aide Training, Certification, and Competency Evaluation Program	1:28	418.94
Hospice/Home Care Volunteers	1:29	418.70
Hospice Patients Residing in Personal Care or Skilled Nursing Facilities	1:30	418.20
Hospice Support Group	1:31	418.70
Incident Reporting	1:32	418.52
Infection Control: Universal Blood and Body Fluid Precaution	1:33	418.66
Infection Control Tracking and Reporting	1:34	418.66
Intake Procedure	1:35	418.82
Interdisciplinary Group	1:36	418.68
Interdisciplinary Group Coordination	1:37	418.58, 418.68
Interdisciplinary Plan of Care	1:38	418.58, 418.68
Letter of Explanation for Funeral Directors	1:39	
Levels of Care	1:40	418.98
Licensure and Certification Verification	1:41	418.72
Medical Device Reporting	1:42	418.96
Medical Services Plan of Care	1:43	418.54, 418.58, 418.68
Medication	1:44	418.96
Nursing Services	1:45	418.82
Occupational Therapy Services	1:46	418.92
Operational Agreement with Pastoral Care	1:47	418.70(f)
Organizational Chart	1:48	418.52
Organizational Mission	1:49	418.52
Orientation/Education	1:50	418.64
Pain and Symptom Management	1:51	418.96(a), 418.96(b)
Patient's Bill of Rights/Responsibilities	1:52	418.62
Physical Therapy Services	1:53	418.92
Program Statement	1:54	418.52
Protocol for Referrals between Hospital and Hospice Program	1:55	418.52
Purpose and Goals of Hospice Program	1:56	418.50, 418.52
Quality Assessment and Improvement Program	1:57	418.66
Quarterly Record Review	1:58	418.66
Release of Information from Records Containing HIV-Related Information	1:59	418.74(b)
Safety Management	1:60	418.66, 418.82
Selection, Orientation, and Evaluation of Personnel	1:61	418.64
Social Work Services	1:62	418.84
Speech Pathology Services	1:63	418.92
Staff Development	1:64	418.64
Support Group	1:65	
Transfer to Other Settings	1:66	418.56
Twenty-Four-Hour Service	1:67	418.50(b)

Policy Name	Policy Number	COP
Utilization Review	1:68	418.66
Verification of Physician's License	1:69	418.52
Violence/Neglect/Abuse	1:70	418.52
Volunteer Recruitment and Retention	1:71	418.70(c)
Volunteer Services	1:72	418.70
Withdrawal of Life-Sustaining Care	1:73	418:62

1:01
ABINGTON MEMORIAL HOSPITAL COMPLIANCE PROGRAM

COMPLIANCE PROGRAM

Commitment to Maintain High Standards

The Compliance Program was designed to ensure that the hospital will consistently maintain high ethical and legal standards as well as comply with all applicable laws and regulations. The Compliance Program encompasses several phases with the key components noted below:

- *Adoption.* The Compliance Program, including the Code of Conduct, has been formally approved by a resolution of the hospital Board of Trustees. Hospital management supports the Compliance Program and will fully implement it.
- *Administration.* The Compliance Program is administered by the Compliance Committee comprised of senior hospital management. The hospital Compliance Officer is responsible for the administration of daily Compliance Program activities.
- *Education.* The hospital expects all employees to be knowledgeable of all applicable laws and regulations and will offer a continuing compliance education program for all affected employees.
- *Monitoring.* The hospital will periodically conduct compliance reviews to ensure adherence to hospital's Code of Conduct and all applicable laws and regulations.

The AMH Employee Hotline

Purpose. The AMH Employee Hotline provides employees of the hospital with a means of reporting any suspected illegal, unethical, or improper activities in confidence and/or anonymously. For guidance of the definition of these types of activities see "When to Call the Hotline."

All calls to the hotline are taken by the compliance officer who will take down the information you provide, investigate it, and, if verified, take appropriate action. A private code is assigned to your call for any follow-up communication.

Why I Should Call. Hospital employees are responsible for ensuring that Abington Memorial Hospital consistently maintains a high ethical standard and is in compliance with all applicable laws and regulations. See "When to Call the Hotline" for applicable listing.

It should be noted that it is a violation of hospital policy to conduct reprisals against any employee who in good faith makes a report to the Employee Hotline. To help us, we ask that you report any incidence of non-compliance first to your immediate supervisor, manager/director, Human Resources Department, or your vice president. If you feel uncomfortable taking any of these approaches, please call the AMH Employee Hotline.

When to call the hotline. The hospital strongly encourages you to call the AMH Employee Hotline when you believe any illegal, unethical, or improper activities need to be reported, investigated, and rectified. As a guideline, please call the hotline if you know of or suspect any violations of the following:

- all provisions of the AMH Code of Conduct
- medical reimbursement laws and regulations
- harassment/discrimination laws
- internal accounting controls

You can also call the hotline even if you're not sure there is a problem and need clarification regarding a legal or ethical concern.

Origin Date: _____
Revised Date: _____
Approved By: _____
Originator: _____
Distribution: _____

1:02
ACCESS TO TERMINAL CARE FUNDS

The Terminal Care Fund may be used for the care of a hospice patient in the event that the patient's insurance does not cover ancillary services, drugs, and equipment. The funds will be used for the following:

- equipment
- drugs/biologicals
- home health aide/homemaker services

If the above criteria are met, final approval for use of the Terminal Care Fund will be at the discretion of the hospice coordinator and director of finance.

Origin Date: _____
Revised Date: _____
Approved By: _____
Originator: _____
Distribution: _____

1:03
ADDENDUM TO CLINICAL RECORDS

1. When hospice patients are admitted to either Abington Memorial Hospital for short-term acute care, or a contracted nursing home for respite care, the clinical records, policies, and procedures of the respective institutions will be followed.
2. Members of the hospice interdisciplinary group who visit the patient in the acute care or skilled nursing facility will have access to the inpatient clinical record for review and documentation.
3. A copy of the interdisciplinary group plan will be placed on the inpatient clinical record. Upon discharge, a detailed summary of the patient's inpatient stay will be sent to hospice along with any additional documentation the hospice requires.

4. Refer to Clinical Record Policy of Abington Memorial Hospital and/or the contracted nursing home. When required for quality assurance review, a copy of the inpatient record will be made available to the hospice.
5. Inpatient records will be reviewed for each hospice patient on an ongoing basis and at discharge to ensure adherence to hospice policies, not to exceed 50 inpatient records per quarter.

Origin Date: _____
Revised Date: _____
Approved Date: _____
Originator: _____
Distribution: _____

1:04
ADDRESSING ETHICAL ISSUES

PURPOSE:

To establish guidelines for staff in addressing ethical issues

RESPONSIBLE PERSONNEL:

Executive director, director of professional services, supervisors, staff and contractors, hospital ethics committee

OBJECTIVES:

- To establish a mechanism for addressing ethical issues arising in the care of patients/clients
- To ensure patient, staff, and physician participation in the consideration of ethical issues arising in the care of patients/clients
- To orient and educate staff on ethical issues
- To establish guidelines for staff in addressing ethical issues

POLICY:

- It is the policy of Abington Memorial Hospital Home Care (AMHHC) that patients and families have the right to participate in discussions concerning ethical issues arising from patient care. This includes ethical issues regarding the withholding or withdrawal of treatment. Patients are informed of these rights in the "Patients Bill of Rights/Responsibilities," which is discussed during the admission visit.
- The staff of the AMHHC subscribes to an ethical nursing practice model in addressing ethical issues (*Journal of Nursing Administration,* Vol. 23, no. 3, March 1993, p. 23). The model adheres to the following principles:
  - Beneficence: (doing good for others)
  - Non-Maleficence: (do no harm)
  - Autonomy: (accountability for practice)
  - Justice: (fair and equitable treatment of all patients, respect for the beliefs and values of others)
  - Fidelity: (faith and trust in others)

- It is recognized that ethical issues are addressed by physicians, staff, contractors, and supervisors in the performance of their daily duties. In the event that the ethical issue cannot be adequately addressed by the patient's physician, AMHHC staff, and the patient/family, the hospital ethics committee is available for consultation.

PROCEDURE:

Action	Rationale
1. Staff address ethical concerns with patient/family, physician, and supervisor. Ethical concerns may be related to the following: • unsafe home situation • lack of or insufficient reimbursement for care • uncooperative or non-compliant patient • abusive patient • no or inadequate support system • care needs that exceed agency resources • family demands for care that contradicts the patient's desires • withholding or withdrawal of treatment	1. Patient/family, staff, home health agency, and physician participate in the consideration of ethical issues. A framework is available to assist staff in the identification of ethical issues.
2. Supervisor addresses concern with agency administration, which solicits information and conferences with staff. Alternatives are discussed, and staff are educated on resources available.	2. A mechanism is in place for the consideration of ethical issues.
3. At the discretion of administration, the issue may be brought to the ethics committee for discussion and consultation.	3. The hospital ethics committee is available for consultation and guidance. It provides a forum for communication and facilitation of the decision-making process.
4. Documentation of conferences are included in the medical record.	4. Documentation is an agency requirement.

Origin Date: _____
Revised Date: _____
Approved Date: _____
Originator: _____
Distribution: _____

1:05
ADMISSION CRITERIA

PURPOSE:

To identify criteria that establish patient eligibility and suitability for admission to hospice.

RESPONSIBLE PERSONNEL:

All professional visiting staff, administrative staff, supervisory staff

OBJECTIVES:

1. To develop admission criteria
2. To provide guidance to staff in their decision making regarding admission of patients to service
3. To establish uniform admission standards

POLICY:

- Hospice is available to patients without regard for disease entity, color, creed, national origin, age, sex, or ability to pay, given that the following criteria are met:
  - Patient's residence is located within the defined geographical area.
  - Signed physician's plan of care and follow-up required is in accordance with organization's policy.
  - The organization has the ability to meet the needs of the patient/family.
  - There is acceptance of the service policies and proposed plan of care by the patient/family.
  - There is ability and willingness on the part of patient/family to participate in patient's interim care between staff's service visits.
  - There is adequate cooperative effort by patient/family to establish safety measures and a plan for medical emergencies.
  - The patient's home situation is conducive to the needed care of the patient. There are provisions for safety of the patient and home care personnel, as well as food, shelter, clothing, and necessary supplies needed by the patient.
  - There is acceptance of the policy for periodic evaluations, which may indicate change in level, frequency of care, and fee establishment or adjustment.
- Patient must be certified as being terminally ill. The client's attending physician attests that the client has a medical prognosis that limits the life expectancy to six months or less. The hospice physician must concur with this certification. These certifications are obtained in writing and become part of the client's medical record (for Medicare hospice benefit patients). Both physicians must sign the certification statements no later than two calendar days after hospice care is initiated. An oral order within two days allows up to eight days to obtain an initial certification in writing.
- A primary care person will sign the *patient consent for care*. This person will assume responsibility for the patient's care 24 hours a day. The primary care person must also be designated as durable power of attorney for hospice patients living alone. If the primary care person chooses to hire someone to help fulfill this responsibility, the primary care person will bear the financial cost of hiring. The caregiver is also responsible for being available to the patient and staff and for instructing substitute caregivers in known procedures and medication schedule to be carried out by the substitute caregiver.

Hospice team will follow general guidelines of home care regarding teaching of nonemployee home attendants.
- Patient will sign the hospice election forms required by the insurance provider in the presence of a hospice team member after explanation of services available, if able. If unable, the patient's representative will sign the election forms. The patient's representative is an individual who has been authorized to elect, revoke, or terminate medical care on behalf of a terminally ill individual who is mentally or physically incapacitated.
- Patients who do not choose to elect their hospice benefit or are not eligible for a hospice benefit may receive AMH home care provided by hospice team members after signing a Patient Consent for Care form for the hospice program.
- Patients on life-extending or life-support measures are not generally considered appropriate for admission to the hospice program. These measures may include the use of ventilators, dialysis and total parenteral nutrition. Patients will be considered on an individual basis by the hospice team.
- The hospice reserves the right to limit admission if financial and personnel resources are not adequate to provide required care.

Origin Date: _____
Revised Date: _____
Approved Date: _____
Originator: _____
Distribution: _____

1:06
ADVANCE DIRECTIVES

PURPOSE:

To ensure compliance with the Patient Self-Determination Act of 1990

RESPONSIBLE PERSONNEL:

Executive director, director of professional services, supervisors, and professional staff

OBJECTIVES:

- To establish policies and procedures to direct staff in complying with the law
- To provide guidance and direction to staff in ascertaining the existence of an advance directive
- To educate staff and the community on issues concerning advance directives

POLICY:

- In compliance with the Patient Self-Determination Act and Pennsylvania state law, it is the policy of the home care department to ascertain whether or not adult* patients being admitted have an advance directive (e.g., living will or durable power-of-attorney for health care). The home care department will provide information to these patients about advance directives and Pennsylvania state laws. The home care department will not

---

*An adult is 18 years of age or older, or an emancipated minor (a minor who has graduated from high school, has married, has been pregnant, or is living away from parent's home and is self-supporting).

condition the provision of care or otherwise discriminate against an individual based on whether or not the individual has executed an advance directive. The home care department chooses not to establish specific limitations on the ability to comply with an advance directive. All cases will be evaluated on an individual basis. Patients may lodge complaints concerning the implementation of the advance directive requirements to the Home Health Agency Hotline (in Pennsylvania, 1-800-222-0989).
- It is the responsibility of the patient's attending physician to be aware of the patient's wishes as outlined in the advance directive and to determine the course of treatment.

PROCEDURES:
1. As part of the nurse's admission assessment prior to the initiation of care, the nurse will determine whether or not patients have an advance directive. This will be done by asking the patient directly. For those patients who are incapacitated at the start of care and are unable to receive information or articulate the presence of an advance directive, the nurse will ask the next of kin, legal guardian, or significant other.
2. The nurse will document the presence of an advance directive in the computer on the Assessment History screen (under DNR specific instructions) and on the health care team form contained in the patient's home folder. If available, a copy of the advance directive is incorporated into the medical record. The content of the advance directive will be documented in the computer under DNR specific instructions. (*NOTE:* This can only be done to the extent that the patient or caregiver is willing to share the information.)
3. It is the responsibility of the patient's attending physician to be aware of the patient's wishes as outlined in the advance directive, to comply with Pennsylvania state law regarding advance directives, and to then determine the course of treatment.** If available, the advance directive will be placed in the medical record.

**Pennsylvania state law indicates that an advance directive becomes operative when a copy is provided to the attending physician and the declarant is determined by the attending physician to be incompetent (lacking sufficient capacity to make or communicate decisions concerning him- or herself) and in a terminal condition or a state of permanent unconsciousness.

4. If the patient does not have an advance directive at the time of admission, the nurse will ask the patient if he or she wants information about advance directives. The nurse will direct the patient to the brochure regarding advance directives provided to every adult patient admitted. This brochure will have the telephone number of the home care department social worker who can assist the patient regarding advance directives. In addition to the brochure, adult patients will be given information regarding Pennsylvania state law on advance directives. This information will be provided by the state of Pennsylvania.
5. As the patient is considering completing an advance directive, he or she will be encouraged to discuss same with his or her attending physician.
6. If at any time after admission the patient wishes information, and/or has the ability to receive information about advance directives, he or she will be provided with the brochure explaining advance directives. Again, the patient will be encouraged to discuss this with the attending physician.
7. Witnessing (two signatures are required) the execution of a living will or durable power of attorney shall be the responsibility of the home care department social worker and a family member or significant other. Home care department nursing staff may witness as well.
8. It is the policy of the Abington Memorial Hospital Home Care Department to honor a patient's advance directive regarding DNR and/or the withdrawal of life-sustaining treatment. A physician's order is required to implement an advance directive. Staff are required to comply with policies for DNR orders with or without an advance directive.
9. The acknowledgment that the patient/family have been informed of their rights under the Patient Self-Determination Act will be included in the Patient Bill of Rights.

10. If a home care nurse, as a matter of conscience, cannot implement an advance directive, the care of the patient will be transferred to another nurse who does not conscientiously object to complying with the advance directive. If, on the basis of conscience, the department cannot implement an advance directive, every effort will be made to transfer the patient to another provider. In the event that this occurs, the following information will be provided to the patient/family:
    - clarification of the differences between the department/hospital's conscientious objection and those raised by the physician
    - a description of the medical condition or procedure affected by the conscientious objection
    - identification of the state law as the legal authority permitting such objection.
11. Community education is provided by the hospital's education department; however, the home care department staff also distribute advance directive information to the community when presenting to community groups such as ElderMed, Kiwanis, Lions Clubs, etc.

Origin Date: _____
Revised Date: _____
Approved By: _____
Originator: _____
Distribution: _____

1:07
AIDS

PURPOSE:

To establish policy and procedures for the provision of care to the AIDS patient with consideration for the safety of staff

RESPONSIBLE PERSONNEL:

All visiting staff, clinical supervisors, administrative staff

OBJECTIVES:

- To establish the agency's position on the acceptance and care of AIDS patients
- To develop procedures for the protection of agency employees from exposure to the AIDS virus
- To provide guidance and direction to staff in providing patient care

POLICY:

The home care agency accepts appropriate referrals on individuals with a diagnosis of AIDS (acquired immune deficiency syndrome). AIDS is now a reportable disease. As per the Pennsylvania State Department of Health, reporting is the responsibility of the diagnosing physician.

The increasing prevalence of HIV increases the risk that health care workers will be exposed to blood from patients infected with HIV especially when blood and body fluid precautions are not followed for all patients. The Centers for Disease Control (CDC) emphasizes the need for health care workers to consider *ALL* patients as potentially infected with HIV and/or bloodborne pathogens and to adhere rigorously to infection-control precautions for minimizing the risk of exposure to blood and body fluids of all patients.

Since medical history and examination cannot reliably identify all patients infected with HIV or other blood-borne pathogens, universal blood and body fluid precautions are recommended for ALL patients.*

PROCEDURE:

ACTION	RATIONALE
1. Gloves must be worn for any direct contact with patient's blood, body fluids, or secretions, as well as when handling soiled items, services, and materials contaminated with blood, body fluids, or stool.	1. To ensure protection of staff from exposure to the virus; to provide protection to the immunosuppressed patient.
2. Gowns are required if there is potential for soilage of caregivers clothing with patient's blood, body fluids, or stool.	2. To ensure protection of staff from exposure to the virus.
3. Masks and goggles are required when performing procedures that may cause blood or body fluids to splash directly onto the face.	3. To prevent exposure to the mucous membranes of the mouth, nose, and eyes.

---

*Centers for Disease Control and Prevention, *Morbidity and Mortality Weekly Report*. "Recommendations for Prevention of HIV Transmission in Health Care Workers," Vol. 36, no. 25, (August 21, 1987): 35–55.

4. Hands must be washed before and after contact with the patient with an antiseptic microbial skin cleanser or immediately if they become contaminated with blood, stool, body fluids, excretions, or secretions.	4. To prevent cross-contamination from caregiver to patient and vice versa; to protect patients/clients with compromised immunity.
5. Ventilation devices must be used when resuscitating a patient.	5. To minimize exposure that may occur during emergency mouth-to-mouth resuscitation.
6. Use all disposable supplies, including syringes, needles, and instruments. Luerlock syringes should be used. Thermometers are provided by the patient/family or by the hospice program and left in the home for use. Vacutainers will be provided for the patient and then discarded after termination of service. *Note:* Extraordinary care must be taken to avoid accidental wounds from sharp instruments contaminated with potentially infectious material.	6. To prevent cross-contamination of blood products from patient to patient; to protect patients/clients with compromised immunity.
7. Soiled articles, dressings, gowns, and gloves should be wrapped in newspaper, tied securely, placed in a bag, and disposed of in a heavy plastic trash bag that is tightly secured.	7. Double wrapping affords protection from exposure by contaminated articles.
8. Needles should *not* be bent, broken, or returned to original sheath. Place in a puncture-resistant container and dispose of according to Disposal of Used Syringes procedure (1:19).	8. To prevent staff from exposure due to accidental needle injury.
9. Excretions and secretions should be promptly flushed down the toilet. Containers should be disposed of as in #7 or soaked in 1:10 dilution of 5.25% sodium hypochlorite (household bleach) and water for 30 minutes.	9. The HIV virus does not withstand exposure to sodium hypochlorite.
10. Blood and other specimens should be placed in a second impervious container and prominently labeled on the outside as "Biohazard." The label should be secured with tape.	10. Staff and lab technicians will be alerted that the specimen may be HIV positive.
11. Containers or vacutainers contaminated with blood, blood spills, or surfaces contaminated with excretions or secretions should be promptly washed with disinfectant (1:10 dilution of household bleach and water).	11. The HIV virus does not withstand exposure to sodium hypochlorite (household bleach).

12. Linen care: a. Soak contaminated linen in 1:10 solution of bleach and water for 30 minutes. b. Then wash separately in home or a laundromat in the usual way.	12. The HIV virus does not withstand exposure to sodium hypochlorite (household bleach).
13. Whenever possible, a separate room is recommended for patients too ill to use good hygiene, such as individuals with profuse diarrhea, incontinence, or behavioral changes secondary to central nervous system infections.	13. To prevent exposure to household members; to enable caregivers to remove themselves from the sick room; to protect patient/client with compromised immunity.
14. Sphygmomanometer should be placed over a dry skin area that has been covered with a layer of material to maintain barrier. The diaphragm of the stethoscope should be cleaned with an alcohol wipe.	14. To maintain cleanliness of equipment.
15. Staff with skin lesions and upper respiratory infections (in transmissible phase) should not be providing service for patients with AIDS.	15. To prevent reverse contamination in immunosuppressed patients. CMV exposure during pregnancy may cause congenital anomalies.

Origin Date: _____
Revised Date: _____
Approved By: _____
Originator: _____
Distribution: _____

1:08
BEREAVEMENT PROGRAM

POLICY:

- Bereavement services are available to survivors for an appropriate period of time up to one year after the death of a patient.
- Survivors are informed of the types of bereavement care and are followed as per individual need and desire.

Characteristics of the Program:

1. Bereavement services include
   - an initial bereavement assessment, which begins at admission and is updated during the course of care, at time of death, and during bereavement follow-up
   - a process of assessment of possible pathological grief reactions and, as needed, referral for intervention
   - an exchange of information between those providing bereavement services and team members who cared for the patient
2. Hospice volunteers who provide bereavement support have completed appropriate training.

3. The bereavement services fall under the supervision of the director of volunteers, who is responsible for bereavement program management and a plan of contacts, in conjunction with the social worker and/or the chaplain, as needed.

Bereavement Follow-Up Process:

1. The team is notified of the patient's death as soon as possible by the hospice nurse or coordinator.
2. The hospice permits one bereavement visit by the professional staff at the funeral, memorial service, or home.
3. During the case conference following the patient's death, special considerations for bereavement follow-up will be discussed, including possible need for referral. Three levels of risk are assigned by the team:
    a. *Low risk:* Normal grief and reconciliation—follow regular bereavement plan.
    b. *Moderate risk:* May need additional support—monitor.
    c. *High risk:* Requires additional support—monitor closely for possible referral and intervention.

    If a hospice patient's family is considered low risk, the assigned volunteer may carry the family through the bereavement period with backup from the director of volunteers.
4. Problems such as pathologic grief will be brought by the volunteer to the director of volunteers and then to the hospice interdisciplinary group for appropriate referral to other resources. Survivors who evidence problems with grieving will be referred to appropriate resources by the hospice interdisciplinary group.
5. A bereavement card will be initiated by the director of volunteers and a plan of contacts determined with the volunteer and the director. A bereavement volunteer is assigned to follow up with the survivor. Contacts with the patient's survivors will be by visit, telephone call, or mail. A sample schedule might be initial assessment at three weeks followed by contacts at 3, 6, and 12 months.
6. Reporting/recordkeeping: A card file will be maintained by the director of volunteers, which will include the plan, schedule, and a brief report of the contact. The initial assessment form shall be completed either during a home visit or through telephone contact by the volunteer. Subsequent contacts may be by telephone. Forms shall be completed by the volunteer and returned to the home care office in a timely fashion. Bereavement records are kept in the volunteer office until discharge at one year after the patient's death, when they will be placed with the clinical record.
7. Grief recovery support group is offered in the fall and spring and is conducted by the director of volunteers. Each program consists of 12 sessions. The bereavement program helps clients understand the grief process and learn effective ways of coping with the emotional responses and common feelings related to the loss of a loved one.
8. Training shall be provided for the bereavement volunteers in usual grief, recovery and bereavement counseling techniques. This in-service training, provided by the director of volunteers, shall consist of 10 two-hour sessions in addition to the hospice volunteer training course.

Origin Date: _____
Revised Date: _____
Approved By: _____
Originator: _____
Distribution: _____

1:09
BYLAWS

ARTICLE 1: PURPOSE

1.1 PURPOSE. The purpose of Abington Memorial Hospital (the "Corporation") is the support and management of an institution for the purpose of affording medical and surgical aid and nursing to sick and disabled persons of every creed, nationality, and color.

ARTICLE II: MEMBERSHIP

2.1 APPOINTMENT AND REMOVAL. The Members of the Corporation shall be those persons who serve from time to time as Trustees of Abington Memorial Health Care Corporation, in each case to serve in such capacity at the discretion of Abington Memorial Health Care Corporation, and subject to removal by Abington Memorial Health Care Corporation at any time with or without cause.

2.2 MEETINGS. The annual meeting of the Members of the Corporation for the purpose of electing the Board of Trustees of the Corporation from among these candidates nominating committee of the Board of Trustees of Abington Memorial Health Care Corporation shall be on the same date as, and shall immediately follow, the annual organizational meeting of the Board of Trustees of Abington Memorial Health Care Corporation. Special meeting of the Members may be called at any time by the Chairman of the Board, the President, at least one-third of the Board of Trustees, or at least one-third of the Members. Meetings of the Members may be held at any place within or without the Commonwealth of Pennsylvania.

2.3 NOTICE. Written notice of the time and place of the annual meeting and all special meetings of the Members shall be mailed or delivered at least five days in advance of the meeting (unless a longer period of notice is required by applicable law, by the Articles of Incorporation, or by these Bylaws), and notice of all special meetings of the Members shall state the general nature of the business to be transacted. Any written notice shall be delivered personally or by mail. If mailed, such notice shall be deemed to be delivered when deposited in the United States mail, postage prepaid, addressed to a Member at such Member's most recent address listed in the records of the Corporation.

2.4 VOTING. Each Member shall be entitled to one vote.

2.5 QUORUM. One-third of the members shall constitute a quorum for the transaction of business at any meeting of the Members, unless a greater proportion is required by applicable law, by the Articles of Incorporation, or by these Bylaws.

ARTICLE III: BOARD OF TRUSTEES

3.1 NUMBER/QUALIFICATIONS. The Board of Trustees (sometimes referred to as the "Board" and individual members thereof referred to as "Trustee" or "Trustees") manage the business and affairs of the Corporation. The Board shall consist of the individuals then serving as the Chairman and Vice Chairman of the Board, the President, Secretary and Treasurer of the Corporation, the Chief of Medical, Dental and Pediatric Staff of the Corporation ("Staff"), the President and First Vice President of the Women's Board of Abington Memorial Health Care Corporation ("Women's Board"), the Chairman of the Board of Abington Memorial Health Care Corporation, and the Life Trustee of the Corporation (the "Life Trustee") (collectively "Ex-Officio Trustees") and such number of additional Trustees as the Members may from time to time determine, but in no case less than ten (10) or more than twenty-seven (27) Trustees in the aggregate excluding Emeritus and Honorary Trustees. Each Trustee must be at least 21 years of age and willing to serve the interests of the Corporation.

3.2 ELECTION AND TERM.

3.2.1 Each Ex-Officio Trustee shall serve as a Trustee by virtue of the office he or she holds. The remaining Trustees shall be elected by the Members as follows:

3.2.1.1 At each annual organizational meeting of the Members such number of Trustees shall be elected by the Members for a term of five years, to fill such vacancies as the Members determine exist.

3.2.2 All Trustees, except the Ex-Offico Trustees, shall serve for a term of five years or until their successors are elected and have qualified. All Ex-Officio Trustees shall serve until they no longer hold their respective offices. Any individual who shall have served as a Trustee for a period of twelve years or more shall, upon written request delivered to the Chairman of the Board, be designated an Emeritus Trustee, and as such, shall have the privilege of receiving notice of and attending meetings of the Board (but without any right to vote at such meetings), of participating in discussions at such meetings and of receiving minutes of such meetings and any written materials distributed by the Board. No Trustee, except the Ex-Officio Trustees, shall succeed him- or herself in office or be eligible for re-election for a period of one year after serving five successive years as a Trustee.

3.2.3 The Board may, from time to time, appoint individuals to the position of Honorary Trustee. Any individual serving in such position shall have the privilege of receiving notice of and attending meetings of the Board (but without any right to vote at such meetings), of participations in discussions at such meetings and of receiving minutes of such meetings and any written materials distributed to Trustees concerning the Corporation.

3.2.4 Any vacancy arising because of the death, resignation, or removal of a Trustee prior to the expiration of his or her five-year term shall not be filled until the next annual organizational meeting of the Members, when a Trustee shall be elected to fill the vacancy for a full five-year term.

3.2.5 All newly elected Trustees shall be provided with an orientation concerning Board functions and procedures.

3.3 MEETINGS. The annual organizational meeting of the Board of Trustees for, among other purposes, the election of officers shall be held on the first Tuesday of November or at such other time and such place as the Board may from time to time determine. Regular meetings of the Board shall be held on the last Tuesday of each month, except during the month of August, or at such other time and place as the Board may from time to time determine. The Board shall designate one meeting each year to be open to the general public. Notice of this open meeting will be placed in at least one local newspaper no later than two weeks before the meeting. Special meetings of the Board may be called at any time by the Chairman of the Board, the President, or not less than one-third of all Trustees. Meetings of the Board of Trustees may be held at any location within or without the Commonwealth of Pennsylvania.

3.4 NOTICE. Written notice of the time and place of all meetings of the Board of Trustees shall be delivered to each Trustee at least five days prior to the date of such meeting (unless a longer period of notice is required by applicable law, by the Articles of Incorporation, or by these Bylaws) and, in the case of special meetings, shall state the general nature of the business to be transacted. Written notice shall be delivered personally or by mail. If mailed, such notice shall be deemed to be delivered when deposited in the United States mail, postage prepaid, addressed to the designated Trustee at such Trustee's most recent address listed in the records of the Corporation.

3.5 QUORUM. One-third of the Trustees then in office shall constitute a quorum for the transaction of business at any meeting of the Board of Trustees, unless a greater proportion is required by applicable law, by the Articles of Incorporation, or by these Bylaws.

3.6 VOTING. Each Trustee, including the Ex-Officio Trustees, shall be entitled to one vote on any matter submitted to a vote of the Board of Trustees. The acts approved by the affirmative vote of a majority of the Trustees present at a meeting at which a quorum is present shall be the acts of the Board a Trustees unless a greater proportion of affirmative votes is required by applicable law, by the Articles of Incorporation, or by these Bylaws.

3.7 CONFLICT OF INTEREST.

3.7.1 Any duality of interest or possible conflict of interest on the part of a Trustee shall be disclosed to the Board of Trustees and made a matter of record.

3.7.2 Any Trustee having a duality of interest or possible conflict of interest on a matter shall not vote or use his or her personal influence on such matter. Such Trustee may, however, be counted in determining a quorum for the meeting at which the matter is voted upon and may state a position on such matter and provide information which may be of value to the Board in its deliberations.

3.8 REMOVAL. Any Trustee may be removed from office at any time, without assigning any cause, by the Members of the Corporation.

3.9 LIMITATION OF LIABILITY. Trustees shall not be personally liable for monetary damages as such for any action taken, or any failure to take action, unless (a) the Trustee has breached or failed to perform the duties of the Trustee's office as set forth under Section 8363 of the Pennsylvania Director's Liability Act; and (b) the breach or failure to perform constitutes self-dealing, willful misconduct, or recklessness. The provisions of this paragraph shall not apply to (a) the responsibility or liability of a Trustee pursuant to any criminal statute; or (b) the liability of a Trustee for the payment of taxes pursuant to local, state, or federal law.

ARTICLE IV: OFFICERS

4.1 OFFICERS GENERALLY; ELECTION. The officers of the Corporation shall be a Chairman of the Board, one or more Vice Chairmen (but in no event more than two), a President, and Executive Vice President, one or more Vice Presidents, a Secretary, and a Treasurer and such other officers as the Board of Trustees deems desirable. Any two or more offices may be held by the same person. In addition to the powers and duties set forth in these Bylaws, each officer shall have such powers and duties as are usually related to his office and as the Board may determine by resolution. All officers shall hold office for a term of one year (or such other term as the Board shall determine for any office from time to time) or until their successors are elected and have qualified.

4.2 CHAIRMAN OF THE BOARD. The Chairman of the Board, who shall be an Ex-Officio Trustee, shall preside at all meetings of the Board of Trustees and shall perform such other duties as may be assigned by the Board. The Chairman shall be an ex-officio member of all Committees, with full right to participate and vote in the proceedings of each such Committee.

4.3 VICE CHAIRMAN. The Vice Chairmen, who shall be Ex-Officio Trustees, shall perform such duties as may be assigned to them by the Board of Trustees or the Chairman of the Board. In the event of a vacancy in the office of Chairman of the Board or during his or her absence or in the event of his or her disability, inability, or refusal to act, the Vice Chairman shall (in the order of their years of service as a Vice Chairman) perform the duties of the Chairman of the Board with full powers of, and subject to the restrictions on, the Chairman.

4.4 PRESIDENT. The President, who shall be an Ex-Officio Trustee, shall be the chief executive officer of the Corporation and shall control and manage the property, business, and affairs of the Corporation, subject to the policies and directions of the Board of Trustees. The President shall be an Ex-Officio member of all Committees, with full right to participate and vote in the proceedings of each such Committee.

4.5 EXECUTIVE VICE PRESIDENT. The Executive Vice President shall assist the President in the performance of official duties and shall perform the duties of the President in the event of the President's absence, incapacity, or death.

4.6 VICE PRESIDENT. The Vice President and/or Vice Presidents shall perform such duties as may be assigned by the Executive Vice President or President.

4.7 SECRETARY. The Secretary, who shall be an Ex-Officio Trustee, shall keep the minutes of all meetings of the Board of Trustees and shall have charge and custody of the seal and records of the Board of the Corporation.

4.8 TREASURER. The Treasurer, who shall be an Ex-Officio Trustee, shall have charge and custody of all funds of the Corporation, shall maintain an accurate accounting system, and shall present financial reports to the Board of Trustees in such manner and form as the Board may from time to time determine.

ARTICLE V: COMMITTEES

5.1 COMMITTEES IN GENERAL.

5.1.1 STANDING COMMITTEES. The Board may, by resolution, establish such Standing Committees of the Board (and in each case appoint the members and the chairman thereof based on the recommendations of the Chairman of the Board) as it deems necessary or desirable ("Standing Committees"), including, without limitation, the Executive Committee described below. All Standing Committees, except the Executive Committee, shall be comprised of Trustees, Trustees of Abington Memorial Health Care Corporation, Trustees of Abington Properties Corporation, or Directors or Trustees of any other affiliate of the Corporation, provided that at least a majority of the members of any such Standing Committee must be Trustees. The Executive Committee shall be comprised of Trustees only. Only a Trustee may serve as Chairman of any Standing Committee. The Chairman of the Board and the President of the Corporation shall be members of all Standing Committees. The Board may delegate such authority to a Standing Committee as it deems appropriate and is not prohibited by applicable law. All Standing Committees and their members shall serve at the discretion of the Board.

5.1.2 SPECIAL COMMITTEES. The Board may, by resolution, establish one or more Special Committees to advise the Board and the President in the performance of their duties ("Special Committees"), including without limitation, the Budget, Personnel/Pension, Professional Affairs, Quality Assessment, Special Hearing, and Trustee Distinguished Service Award Committees described below. No Special Committee may have or exercise any authority of the Board to manage the business and affairs of the Corporation. All Special Committees and their members shall serve at the discretion of the board.

5.1.3 TERM. Each member of a Standing or Special Committee shall continue as such until the next annual organizational meeting of the Board of Trustees and until a successor has been appointed and has qualified unless sooner removed or unless such committee is sooner dissolved by the Board.

5.1.4 QUORUM. One-third of the members of a Standing or Special Committee shall constitute a quorum for the transaction of any business, and the acts of the majority of the committee members present shall be the acts of such committee in each case, unless a greater proportion is required by applicable law, by the Articles of Incorporation or by these Bylaws.

5.1.5 VACANCIES AND REMOVAL. Vacancies in membership of any committee may be filled by appointments made in the same manner as provided in the case of the original appointments. Any member of a committee may be removed at any time by the Board of Trustees, with or without cause.

5.2 EXECUTIVE COMMITTEE.

5.2.1 The Executive Committee shall consist of the Chairman of the Board, the President, and at least five other trustees.

5.2.2 The Executive Committee shall have and exercise the authority of the Board of Trustees, to the extent permitted by applicable statute, subject to Section 5.2.3 between meetings of the Board, including the following:

5.2.2.1 reviewing and advising on the coverage and insured amounts under the various casualty and liability insurance policies covering the Corporation.

5.2.3 The Executive Committee shall not have the authority of the Board of Trustees with respect to the following matters:

5.2.3.1 amending, altering, or repealing these Bylaws;

5.2.3.2 electing, appointing, or removing any member of the Executive Committee or any Trustee or officer of the Corporation;

5.2.3.3 amending the Articles of the Incorporation;

5.2.3.4 adopting a plan of merger or adopting a plan of consolidation with another corporation;

5.2.3.5 authorizing the sale, lease, exchange, or mortgage of all or substantially all of the property and assets of the Corporation;

5.2.3.6 authorizing the voluntary dissolution of the Corporation or revoking proceedings;

5.2.3.7 adopting a plan for the distribution of the assets of the Corporation.

5.2.4 Meetings of the Executive Committee may be called at any time by the Chairman of the Committee or by any two members of the Committee. Written notice of special meetings of the Executive Committee shall be given at least two days before such meeting.

5.2.5 Minutes of all Executive Committee meetings shall be prepared and presented to the Board of Trustees for review at the next regular meeting of the Board.

5.3 BUDGET COMMITTEE.

5.3.1 The Budget Committee shall consist of such individuals as the Board deems appropriate.

5.3.2 The Budget Committee shall be responsible for reviewing the proposed annual operating and capital budgets of the Corporation and making recommendations relating to such budgets to the Board.

5.4 PERSONNEL/PENSION COMMITTEE.

5.4.1 The Personnel/Pension Committee shall consist of four or more members, including at least four Trustees, including the President of the Corporation or his designee.

5.4.2 The Personnel/Pension Committee shall recommend policies concerning the employees of the Corporation, including fringe benefits and employee relations. The committee also shall advise the executive Committee or the Board of Trustees with respect to the administration and interpretation of any pension or other employee benefit plan maintained by the Corporation. The Personnel/Pension Committee shall report to the Board.

5.5 PROFESSIONAL AFFAIRS COMMITTEE.

5.5.1 The Professional Affairs Committee shall consist of seven or more members, including at least six Trustees, including the President of the Corporation.

5.5.2 The Professional Affairs Committee shall:

5.5.2.1 receive recommendations from the Staff and make final recommendations to the Board on all appointments to, and assignments of responsibilities within, the Staff;

5.5.2.2 recommend to the Board the privileges to be granted to each member of the Staff;

5.5.2.3 recommend to the Board Staff rules and regulations for the government of the Staff, or amendments thereto, necessary to ensure the proper care of the patients;

5.5.2.4 receive and make recommendations to the Board concerning any communications, requests, or recommendations presented by the Staff through duly authorized representatives, including matters concerned with the professional education of the house staff;

5.5.2.5 recommend to the Board specific actions in response to Staff executive committee recommendations/requests for the purpose of and replacement of equipment utilized in care of patients.

5.5.3 The presence in person of a majority of the members of the Professional Affairs Committee shall constitute a quorum for the transaction of business at any meeting of the Committee.

5.5.4 Minutes of all Professional Affairs Committee meetings shall be prepared and presented to the Board of Trustees for review at the next regular meeting of the Board.

5.6 QUALITY ASSESSMENT.

5.6.1 The Quality Assessment Committee shall consist of at least eleven members, including the President of the Corporation, the Chief of Staff, the Chairman of the Professional Affairs Committee, President of the Staff, the Chairman of the Utilization Review Committee of the Staff, the Vice President for Patient Care and Quality Assurance, and the Chairman of the Department of Nursing or his or her designee and at least two other Trustees. The Vice President for Patient Care and Quality Assurance of the Corporation and the Chief of Staff shall serve as co-chairmen.

5.6.2 The Quality Assessment Committee shall establish and maintain a program of quality assessment complying with the standards of the Joint Commission on Accreditation of Healthcare Organizations and other standards established by the Corporation.

5.6.3 Minutes of all Quality Assessment Committee meetings shall be prepared and presented to the Professional Affairs Committee.

5.7 SPECIAL HEARING COMMITTEE.

5.7.1 The Special Hearing Committee shall consist of eleven members: the President of the Corporation or his or her designee, the Chief of Staff, the President of the Staff, three additional members of the Staff, and five additional members of the Board of Trustees. The members of the Staff shall be elected by the staff to serve for a term of two years. The members of the Board shall be appointed annually by the Board Chairman. Vacancies of elected or appointed members shall be filled by the Chief of Staff or Chairman of the Board, respectively, until successors have been elected or appointed. One of the Board members shall be appointed by the Board to serve as Chairman of the Committee.

5.7.2 The Special Hearing Committee shall be responsible for conducting hearings and taking such other action in performing such other duties as contemplated under the Staff bylaws in connection with corrective action and matters affecting Staff membership or privileges generally.

5.8 TRUSTEE DISTINGUISHED SERVICE AWARD COMMITTEE.

5.8.1 The Trustee Distinguished Service Award Committee shall consist of such individuals as the Board deems appropriate.

5.8.2 The Trustee Distinguished Service Award Committee shall be responsible for identifying and recommending individuals who are appropriate candidates for service awards.

ARTICLE VI: MEDICAL, DENTAL, AND PODIATRIC STAFF

6.1 APPOINTMENT.

6.1.1 The Board of Trustees shall appoint a Medical, Dental, and Podiatric Staff ("the Staff") consisting of physicians, dentists, and podiatrists who shall be graduates of recognized medical, dental, or podiatric schools, shall require that they be organized in a responsible administrative body, and that they adopt bylaws, rules, and regulations for the government of their practice in the Corporation's hospital. The bylaws and all hospitalwide rules and regulations for governing the Staff shall be subject to approval by the Board in the exercise of its responsibilities to the patients of the hospital. Persons duly appointed to the Staff shall have full authority and responsibility for the care of patients, subject only to such limitations as the Board may impose, to these Bylaws, and to the bylaws and rules and regulations of the Staff.

6.1.2 All applications for appointments to the Staff shall be in writing and addressed to the Chief of Staff. The applications shall require full information on the prescribed application form concerning the applicant's education, licensure, practice, previous hospital experience, any unfavorable history with regard to licensure and hospital privileges, and any other information as may be required by the bylaws of the Staff. All such applications shall be referred by the Chief of Staff for review to the Board as provided in the bylaws of the Staff.

6.1.3 All appointments to the Staff shall be for a provisional period of one year. Reappointment beyond that term shall be based upon reappraisal of the practitioner as determined in the bylaws of the Staff. When an appointment is not to be renewed or when privileges have been or are proposed to be reduced, altered, suspended, or terminated, the Staff member shall be entitled to an appeal as provided in the bylaws of the Staff.

6.2 DUTIES.

6.2.1 The Board of Trustees shall, in the exercise of its overall responsibility, assign to the Staff reasonable authority for ensuring appropriate professional care to the hospital's patients.

6.2.2 The Staff shall conduct an ongoing review and appraisal of the quality of professional care rendered in the hospital and shall report such activities and their results to the Board of Trustees.

6.2.3 The Staff shall make recommendations to the Board of Trustees concerning: (1) appointments, reappointments, and other changes in Staff status; (2) granting of clinical privileges; (3) all matters relating to professional competency; and (4) such specific matters as may be referred to it by the Board.

6.3 STAFF BYLAWS. The bylaws and rules and regulations of the Staff setting forth its organizations and government shall be recommended by the Staff, and such bylaws and rules and regulations shall be effective when approved by the Board of Trustees. Such bylaws and rules and regulations, and any amendment thereto, shall be binding on all members of the Staff. The Staff shall have the initial responsibility to formulate, adopt, and recommended to the Board Staff bylaws, and amendments thereto, which shall be effective when approved by the Board. If the staff fails to exercise this responsibility in good faith and in a reasonable, timely, and responsible manner, and after written notice from the Board to such effect, including a reasonable period of time for response, the Board may resort to its own initiative in formulating or amending Staff bylaws. In such event, Staff recommendations and views shall be carefully considered by the Board during its deliberations and in its actions.

ARTICLE VII: CHIEF OF STAFF

7.1. CHIEF OF STAFF. The Board of Trustees shall appoint and fix the compensation of a Chief of Staff whose services shall continue at the pleasure of the Board.

ARTICLE VIII: INDEMNIFICATION

8.1 RIGHT TO INDEMNIFICATION. The Corporation shall indemnify any person who was or is a party or threatened to be made a party to any threatened, pending, or completed action, suit, or proceeding, whether civil, criminal, administrative, or investigative, by reason of the fact that such person (a) is or was a Trustee, employee, or officer (including assistant officer) of the Corporation; or (b) is or was serving in an administrative capacity, including as a Department Chairman or Division Chief or on a Committee of the Staff or of the Corporation, including the Special Hearing Committee, in their respective administrative functions, pursuant to the Staff or Corporation bylaws; or (c) is or was serving at the request of the Corporation or the Staff on a Review Organization as that term is defined in the Pennsylvania Peer Review Protection Act (or any successor statute) and exercised due care in that capacity; or (d) is or was serving, at the request of the Corporation, as a Trustee, officer, employee, or agent of another organization; or (e) is or was a Trustee, officer, or the employee or agent of the Corporation serving at its request as an administrator, Trustee, or other fiduciary of one or more of the Corporation's employee benefit plans, against expenses (including attorney's fees), judgments, fines, excise taxes, and amounts paid in settlement actually and reasonably incurred by such person in connection with such action, suit, or proceeding whether or not the indemnified liability arises or arose from any threatened, pending, or completed action by or in the right of the Corporation, to the extent that such person is not insured or otherwise indemnified and except as prohibited by statute. For this purpose and for the purposes of Section 8.2 below, the Board may, and on request of any such person shall be required to, determine in each case whether or not any applicable statutory standards have been met, or such determination shall be made by independent legal counsel if the Board so directs or if the Board is not empowered by statute to make such determination.

8.2 ADVANCE EXPENSES. Expenses incurred by Trustee, officer, or employee in defending a civil or criminal action, suit, or proceeding shall be paid by the Corporation in advance of the final disposition of such action, suit, or proceeding upon receipt of an undertaking by or on behalf of the trustee, officer, or employee to repay such amount if it shall ultimately be determined that such person is not entitled to be indemnified by the Corporation.

8.3 INDEMNIFICATION NOT EXCLUSIVE. The foregoing indemnification shall not be deemed exclusive of any other right to which one indemnified may be entitled, both as to action in such person's official capacity and as to action and another capacity while holding such office, and shall inure to the benefit of the heirs, executors, and administrators of any such person.

8.4 INSURANCE AND OTHER INDEMNIFICATION. The Board of Trustees shall have the power (a) to purchase and maintain, at the Corporation's expense, insurance on behalf of the Corporation and on behalf of others to the extent that power to do so has been or may be granted by statute, and (b) to give other indemnification to the extent not prohibited by law.

ARTICLE IX: MISCELLANEOUS

9.1 FISCAL YEAR. The fiscal year of the Corporation shall begin on the first day of July and shall end on the 30th day of June.

9.2 AUDIT. The Board of Trustees shall select an independent public accountant or accountants to make an audit of the books and accounts of the Corporation for each fiscal year.

9.3 POLICIES AND PROCEDURES. The Board shall establish policies and procedures for implementing, disseminating, and enforcing a Patient's Bill of Rights; orienting new Board members; offering continuing education to Board members; periodically reexamining the relationship of the Board to the community; and adopting such other policies and procedures as the Board may, from time to time, determine to be appropriate or desirable.

ARTICLE X: AMENDMENTS

10.1 REVIEW. The Members and the Board shall review these Bylaws at least once every year and shall make revisions as necessary in accordance with Section 10.2 below, indicating the date or dates when last reviewed and revised.

10.2 AMENDMENTS. These Bylaws may be altered, amended, or repealed or new Bylaws may be adopted by the Board of Trustees at any meeting of the board by the vote of not less than two-thirds of the Trustees present at any such meeting or by the members of the Corporation at any meeting of Members by the vote of not less than two-thirds of the Members present at any such meeting, provided that notice of any proposed amendment or a summary thereof shall have been given to each Trustee or Member not less than ten days prior to the date of the meeting and, provided further, that in each case any such alteration, amendment, or repeal shall not become effective until the approval of Abington Memorial Health Care Corporation is obtained.

Origin Date: _____
Revised Date: _____
Approved By: _____
Originator: _____
Distribution: _____

1:10
CLINICAL RECORDS

PURPOSE:

To ensure the availability of clinical data and information necessary for the provision of hospice services in a systematic and confidential manner

RESPONSIBLE PERSONNEL:

Executive director, director of professional services, supervisors, professional and contract staff, clinical information staff and billing department

OBJECTIVES:

- To maintain a complete clinical record for each patient that provides a history and plan of care for the patient and provides a paper record of all care provided to the patient
- To provide a system for storage and maintenance of all records
- To ensure the confidentiality, security, and integrity of patient information
- To provide standardization of abbreviations, acronyms, symbols, codes, and classification to ensure consistent interpretation of information

POLICY:

- A clinical record is maintained for each patient admitted in an individual folder filed in a color-coded numeric system. Clinical records of current patients and closed records (for approximately one year) are kept in the medical record department in protected files. An additional three to four years of closed records are stored in a secured storage room in the building. All other records are stored off the premises in a storage facility that meets legal requirements. The entire building is fire protected by a sprinkler system.
- For patients receiving acute inpatient care at AMH, the clinical record is maintained at the hospital and forwarded to the home care department at discharge. The home care department will maintain original consent forms, original plan of treatment (POT) form, master file, and discharge information.
- Records are retained for a minimum of seven years in a protected area to safeguard against loss or unauthorized use. Records of minors are retained until the age of majority plus an additional seven years.
- Information from the clinical record will not be disclosed without the patient's consent, except as necessary to provide services and to obtain payment for those services, or in response to a valid subpoena or court order. (See Release of Information from Records Containing HIV-Related Information, 1:59.)
- The final responsibility for patient records rests with the executive director and the governing body. If the organization is dissolved, the State Department of Health will be notified of the date of dissolution and location of the records.

PROCEDURE:

Action	Rationale
Open Records	
1. A clinical record is initiated on every patient admitted for service and a patient number is assigned. The same number is retained for patients readmitted.	1. Accurate information is captured for every patient upon admission and a number is assigned for efficiency in filing all subsequent forms.
2. Open records are filed numerically in the office on a central file maintained by the clinical information staff. Records are filed by straight numeric system, color coded for each 100 records, and for every 10 within the 100.	2. Central files by number and color code provides for optimum efficiency in filing and retrieving information. Central control of files maintains optimum standardization.
3. The contents of the clinical record contain past and current data, as follows: a. *Master file input data:* Contains appropriate identifying information and physician's name and telephone number. • Form is taken on home visits and becomes a permanent part of the record on discharge.	3. The clinical record contains all data on the patient to guide the care by all disciplines while a patient of the hospice services.

- A duplicate copy of the form is kept in the clinical record or supervisor's folder while individual is a patient.
b. *Therapy and medical social service assessment forms:*
    - Contain pertinent past findings and a current clinical assessment of patient's status
    - Completed on admission and readmission
c. *Nursing assessment forms:*
    - Contains pertinent family information
    - Contains pertinent past findings and a current clinical assessment of patient's status
    - Completed on admission and readmission
    - Contains list of nursing diagnosis for each individual problem
d. *Clinical notes:*
    - Current progress notes dated and signed
    - Clinical notes segregated on colored paper for ease in identification of disciplines
e. *Physicians plan of treatment:*
    - Contains a summary report to the physician completed on admission and every 62 days thereafter or as required by individual's insurance coverage (i.e., Medicare hospice benefit)
    - Additions or changes in the POT confirmed with a verbal order
f. *Patient authorization and release form*
g. *Medication list:*
    - Computerized form listing name of medication, dosage, frequency, and route, indications, side effects, and interactions
    - Completed on admission and updated as needed
h. *Discharge summary:*
    - Hospice benefit records have one discharge summary completed by the registered nurse

- Discharge summary includes a summary of service from admission through discharge, including goal attained
  i. *Written communications:* Includes conference reports and reports to and from other participating organizations and to and from multidisciplinary professional personnel
  j. *Home health aid plan of care:* When applicable
  k. *Home health aid activity records:* When applicable
  l. *Patient discharge instruction sheet:*
     - Completed at time of discharge for patients discharged for reasons other than death or transfer to another facility
     - Original to patient and copy in chart
  m. *Patient bill of rights:* Signed copy
  n. *Respite services:* If patient receives inpatient respite services, a discharge summary of services shall be routinely provided to the hospice and a copy of the inpatient record will be available if requested.
4. All records are kept in a standardized file. For patients receiving routine hospice services, the filing sequence is as follows:
   Left side—Front to back
   a. Master File Input (MFI) Card (at discharge)
   b. Verbal orders
   c. Interdisciplinary Care Plan (orders), including (if available)
      - IDG POC for continuous care nursing
      - IDG POC for inpatient respite
      - IDG POC for acute inpatient services
   d. MD Certification of Terminal Illness—Medicare or MA
   e. Election of Hospice—Medicare Benefit or MA
   f. Hospice Program Patient Consent for Care—*All charts*

4. Standardization increases efficiency of filing and retrieving information.

g. Consent for Release of Information—*All charts*
h. Evaluation forms (MSW, PT, OT, ST)
i. Spiritual Assessment
j. Advanced Directive (if available)
k. Home Health Aide POC, including POC for respite shift (if available)
l. Volunteer Assessment and Plan
m. Referral for Services (if available)
n. Authorization and Release—Copy from home care record
o. Bill of Rights—Copy from home care record
p. Home Health Aide Activity Records
q. Miscellaneous—Lab reports, faxes, Hospice Change in Level of Care form.

Right side—Front to back
a. Patient Master Update I (PMUI) (following discharge)
b. Revocation of Hospice Care (Medicare or MA, if available)
c. Change of Designated Hospice (Medicare or MA, if available)
d. Discharge Summary
e. Progress Notes (newest on top):
   - Yellow—Nursing
   - Pink—Physical therapy
   - Gold—Occupational therapy
   - Blue—Speech therapy
   - Green—Social service
   - White—Chaplain
   - Cream—Volunteers
f. Flow Sheets
g. Medication List
h. Nutrition Assessment
i. Braden Pressure Ulcer Risk Assessment
j. Nursing Assessment—Copy from home care chart

5. For patients receiving only acute inpatient services, the AMH record is forwarded to hospice at discharge. This filing sequence is as follows:
   a. *Home care record* (right side):
      - PMUI
      - Nursing Discharge Summary
      - MFI
      - Signed Interdisciplinary Care Plan (orders)

5. Standardization increases efficiency of filing and retrieving information.

- MD Certificate of Terminal Illness (MDA/MA only)
- Election of Hospice Benefit—Medicare only
- Hospice Program Consent for Care
- Release of Information Consent
- Authorization and Release form
- Bill of Rights and Patient Responsibilities
- Medicare Secondary/Payer information

b. *Inpatient record* (left side):
- Death Certificate
- Anatomical Donation
- Front Index Sheet
- Inpatient Face Sheet
- MD D/C Summary
- ER Record (if applicable)
- Progress Notes/Consults
- Clinical Notes (medications)
- Valuable Property Record
- Condition of Admission (if available)
- Vital signs records
- IV records (if available)
- Written/computer orders
- Standards Documentation Flow Sheet
- IDG Patient Database
- Election of Hospice Benefit (copy)
- Hospice Program Consent for Care (copy)
- Release of Information Consent (copy)
- Living Will
- Authorization and Release form (copy)
- Interdisciplinary Care Plan (orders)
- Referral for Services
- Nursing Assessment
- Braden/Nutrition Assessments
- MSW Assessment Form
- MSW Plan of Care
- Volunteer Care Plan
- Volunteer Visit Records

6. The clinical record is combined at discharge for patients who receive both routine and acute inpatient hospice services.

6. Standardization increases efficiency of filing and retrieving information.

a. Home care documentation is combined on the right side of the record.
b. AMH clinical record is filed on the left side.
7. Visiting staff tape records notes after each visit and sends tape with (pink) copy of the Daily Report Sheet to the transcriptionist daily through interoffice mail.
8. The transcriptionist types the notes and returns them to the sender for reading and signature.
9. The professional staff send completed notes to the medical records staff for filing in the patients record on a timely basis.
10. The medical records staff are responsible for maintaining all clinical record supplies in sufficient quantity.

7. Taping results of the visit increases efficiency of visiting staff and increases readability of the stored record.

8. The signature of the professional staff person ensures accuracy of typed note.

9. Filing by the medical records staff saves the time of the professional staff.

10. Supplies are always available as needed.

Reopening a Previous Admission

1. The data of the previous admission are transferred to the right side of the file.
2. The divider is placed on the right side of the file with the tab labeled.
3. Subsequent filing sequence follows current admission order as above.

1. Having the data available from the previous admission is helpful in planning current care for the readmitted patient.
2. Having the data available from the previous admission is helpful in planning current care for the readmitted patient.
3. Having the data available from the previous admission is helpful in planning current care for the readmitted patient.

Discharged Records

1. When a patient is discharged, the order of the file remains the same.
2. The master file input card is placed on the left side.
3. The patient master update discharge form is placed on the right side.
4. The record is filed in the closed record file and kept there for the current year plus one year.
5. Closed records for previous years are stored off the premises in storage that

1. The record is kept intact in case the data are needed for future admissions or other reasons.
2. The record is kept intact in case the data are needed for future admissions or other reasons.
3. The record is kept intact in case the data are needed for future admissions or other reasons.
4. Closed records that need to be accessed are most often within this time frame of discharge.
5. Records are still available if needed but are not using valuable office space.

6. Records are maintained for a minimum of seven years. Records of minors are retained until the patient's age of majority and an additional seven years.

6. Record retention meets hospice and statutory requirements.

Record Documentation

1. All entries into the clinical record must be dated, authenticated, and titled. If the names appear once in the document, initials may be used.
    a. The following staff are authorized to make entries on review in the clinical record: Executive Director, director of professional services, clinical supervisors, home care nurses, therapist (PT, OT, ST), volunteers (hospice), volunteer director (hospice), physicians, therapy clerk, homemaker/home health aide supervisors, volunteer director/assistant coordinator, billing staff, clinical information staff, pastoral care staff (hospice), medical social worker, director of finance, transcriptionists, clinical educator, clinical link trainer/analyst, home health aide clerk, students, home health aides (home health aide activity records only)
    b. The following are authorized to review the medical record: PAC (professional advisory committee) and surveyors from licensing, certification, and accrediting bodies

1. Documentation must be identified to meet legal requirements.

2. All entries recorded in the record must be legible and accurate. Errors are to be corrected but not obliterated. For errors noticed immediately, a line is to be drawn through the material, the correction initialed, and ME (mistaken entry) written above. For errors noted at a later date, the author must write, "There is an error in my note of (date)." Then the note is rewritten at that point in the record, dated with the current date, and signed.

2. All data must be legally acceptable as to accuracy eligibility.

3. Only approved symbols and abbreviations are used in the clinical record and there must be an explanatory legend avail-

3. To prevent misinterpretation, only approved symbols and abbreviations are used.

able to personnel authorized to make and read the entries.

4. A supervisor or another nurse may cosign a document. Cosignature of documents will include the name of the author (i.e., the individual who provided the care) of the document followed by the name or initials of the person who cosigned the document.

4. The nurse or therapist who provided the care is ultimately responsible for the care provided and the content of the documentation.

5. Diagnoses are classified according to the International Classification of Diseases.

5. Acceptable standard of practice.

Confidentiality of Records

1. The confidentiality of the medical record will be maintained. Patients will be instructed to maintain confidentiality of any portion of the record that is left in the home (i.e., home health aide plan of care).

1. It is the responsibility of the department to maintain confidentiality of the medical record to ensure compliance with the Conditions of Participation.

Protection of Records

1. Authorized personnel, including students, volunteers, and cleaning service employees, have access to the clinical information department.

1. Students are accepted upon recommendation of the educational facility. They are required to sign a statement of confidentiality. Selected volunteers are assigned to the department to staff. Cleaning service staff are employees of AMH. Background information on personnel is contained in the personnel department.

2. The clinical information department is secured with locked doors and is fire protected with sprinklers.

2. The agency complies with Medicare regulations.

3. Building complies with municipal fire regulation codes.

3. The agency complies with local ordinances.

Release of Medical Records

1. In response to a subpoena, all portions of the record may be copied.

1. Subpoenas mandate the release of information. Copies of the record are generally acceptable.

2. In response to a request from a governmental insurer and third-party payer, clinical documents may be copied.

2. Government regulations and third-party insurers require release of clinical information to ascertain compliance with regulations and contract specifications also necessary for reimbursement.

3. Staff may copy any portion of the record to facilitate coordination of care.

3. The staff maintain responsibility for the confidentiality for all copies.

4. Copies of the record must be discarded at the home care department.

4. The agency ensures confidentiality of patient care documents.

Use of Computer Mail Documentation

1. The transmission of data via the e-mail system is acceptable for entry into the medical record.

1. Allows for immediate access and retrieval of off-site data.

2. Home health aide schedules or changes will be accepted via the e-mail system.

2. Facilitates coordination of contracted home health aide services.

3. The computerized printout of the change is signed by the individual who takes the message off the computer and enters it into the record.

3. Provides for immediate notification to staff of home health aide changes.

Completion of Record

1. Discharged documentation must be completed within 30 days.
2. The home care record of a patient/client discharged from service is completed within one year.

2. The clinical information department reviews all discharge records for completeness.

Origin Date: _____
Revised Date: _____
Approved By: _____
Originator: _____
Distribution: _____

1:11
COMMUNICATION THROUGH LANGUAGE INTERPRETERS

PURPOSE:

To ensure that patients who speak a non-English language receive full service

RESPONSIBLE PERSONNEL:

Pastoral care department, human resources, and patient relations departments; home care department professional staff

OBJECTIVES:

To provide language interpreters for patients who speak a language other than English

POLICY:

It is recognized by the organization that good communication is essential to foster quality patient care. Thus, every effort is made to provide language interpreters as required by the patient.

PROCEDURE:

Action

Rationale

1. The pastoral care department, together with the human resources and patient relations departments will be responsible for maintaining the sign and foreign language interpreters list. As a supplement, a 24-hour telephone "Language Line" Link has been established for virtually every foreign language. (Optimal communication should be achieved through in-person interpreters when possible.) The home care department, having direct patient responsibility, has information for contacting the service. The pastoral care and patient relations departments will serve as a general guide for access to interpreters. The patient relations or pastoral care department may be contacted during office hours to inquire about the resources for a particular language, including sign language. After office hours, the on-call chaplin may be paged through the hospital operator, and he or she will secure the needed information from the pastoral care office. The home care department will be responsible for contacting the resource. As much advance notice as possible is required to secure the most appropriate resource.

1. Every effort is made to facilitate appropriate care and communication for all patients, including patients whose care may be hindered by a language barrier.

Origin Date: _____
Revised Date: _____
Approved Date: _____
Originator: _____
Distribution: _____

1:12
COMMUNICATION WITH VISUALLY OR HEARING IMPAIRED PATIENTS

PURPOSE:

To ensure that patients with visual or hearing impairments receive full-service

RESPONSIBLE PERSONNEL:

Director of professional services, professional staff, pastoral care, patient relations department

OBJECTIVES:

To formulate and implement procedures to ensure that patients with visual or hearing impairments are not denied effective notice of benefits, waivers of rights, or consent to treat

POLICY:

It is the intent of the organization to fully inform all patients of benefits, rights, and consent to treat, and the agency therefore has established special procedures to ensure same with patients who have either visual or hearing impairments that could interfere with the informed consent process.

PROCEDURE:

Action	Rationale
Visually Impaired Patient	
1. The assigned professional will read aloud all documents normally provided to the patient and ascertain that the person has heard and understands what was read. The professional documents this process on the patient record.	1. Reading to and feedback from the patient ensures that the patient has a reasonable understanding of the document.
2. The assigned professional will make available for the patient's use any large-print patient information that may be applicable to the patient's disease process (e.g., colostomy or diabetic care).	2. This enhances the patient's understanding of his or her condition.
Hearing Impaired Patient	
1. The assigned professional interviewing the patient ascertains the patient's preferred method of communication (i.e.,	1. This allows the patient to participate as fully as possible in his or her care.

paper and pencil, lip reading, sign language).
2. If the preferred method is sign language, the professional contacts the pastoral care or patient relations department, which will provide a list of certified sign language interpreters.
3. The following telecommunication devices for the deaf are available for use by the agency:
   - _____
   - _____

2. Full use is made of all hospital departments to enhance the care to the greatest possible extent.

3. Full use is made of all available community resources to enhance the care to the greatest possible extent.

Origin Date: _____
Revised Date: _____
Approved Date: _____
Originator: _____
Distribution: _____

1:13
COMPETENCY EVALUATION PROGRAM

PURPOSE:
To provide guidelines to agency personnel in complying with the departmental competency evaluation program

RESPONSIBLE PERSONNEL:
Clinical educator, director of quality improvement, director of professional services, director of finance, clinical supervisors, and staff

OBJECTIVES:
- To develop a competency evaluation program in compliance with Joint Commission standards
- To implement a competency program
- To educate all levels of personnel on agency standards and expectations
- To ensure staff's continued ability to perform their respective job functions
- To collect and analyze data to assess staff competence and pinpoint training needs

POLICY:
- It is the policy of AMHHC to ensure that staff are competent to provide professional services and home health aide services to our patient population. It is our expectation that the medical records, billing, information services, and clerical staff support the overall goals of our programs and services by demonstrating competence in their respective functions.

- Our competency program will be a three-step process consisting of entry-level competencies, postorientation/probationary competencies and annual competencies. The program interfaces with the criteria-based performance appraisal system and in part forms a basis on which to evaluate staff.
- Entry-level competencies are defined as those measures of behavior that prudent persons would deem necessary for entry into employment based on the job description (i.e., graduation, verification of licensure, references, competency self-assessment form). Orientation/probationary competencies are competencies that ensure that staff can function safely and competently on a home visit. Such things as infection control, safety, computerized documentation, communications, coordination, hemoccult, chemstrip, and blood glucose monitoring are addressed. In addition, skills that the individual identifies as areas of weakness are also addressed.
- Annual competencies are unit specific and involve being able to demonstrate cognitive and/or psychomotor skills to care for a particular patient population or to perform a specific job function.
- The quality improvement program—through analysis of quality indicator data and identification of high-risk, problem-prone, low-volume, and high-volume areas—enables the administrative and supervisory staff to collect and aggregate data on staff competencies. This analysis, in addition to an ongoing assessment of staff needs (staff education committee, supervisors' meetings, quality council meetings, informal discussion) facilitate the identification of annual competencies. The development and implementation of new clinical guidelines may also form a basis on which to competency test staff.
- For staff and contractors (nursing, PT, OT, MSW), the clinical educator/supervisor or designee will validate annual competencies yearly. Home health aides will be validated annually as part of the performance appraisal system.
- Managers' competencies are validated as part of the annual performance appraisal process. The performance appraisal evaluates affective and cognitive skills. Affective skills are defined as a measure of decision-making ability. They include the attributes of critical thinking, decision making based on pertinent data, and effective communication. Cognitive skills are defined as a measure of knowledge and/or perceptions.
- Certification is encouraged for all levels of staff, as certification deems competence.

PROCEDURE:

Action	Rationale
1. Personal interviews are conducted with all staff, contractors, and volunteers. Interviews allow for the verification of education, experience, training, and certification. Written and/or oral references are obtained to the best of the agency's ability; however, many employees will only verify employment dates. When staff transfer from the hospital, an oral reference is obtained from the manager. Hospital policy does not allow for trans-	1. Reference checks are performed to meet hospital policy as well as Joint Commission and Medicare Conditions of Participation requirements.

fer if an employee is under disciplinary action.
2. Licensure is verified by calling the appropriate licensure board. All other certificates and credentials are requested for inclusion in the personnel file.
3. Nurses, therapy contractors, and social workers complete a competency self-assessment form (skills checklist) during orientation.
4. Throughout the orientation, the clinical educator/supervisor will competency test staff and contractors (nursing, PT, OT, HHA, MSW) on selected basic skills.
5. The clinical educator reviews the skills checklist for areas of weakness. When indicated, skills will be demonstrated in the skills lab. Home visits for competency testing of skills will be scheduled by the supervisor. A nurse experienced in the procedure, the clinical educator, or a nurse practitioner may observe the return demonstration. Supervisors annually review the skills checklist to ascertain learning needs.
6. The clinical educator or the supervisor conducts a home visit to assess knowledge and to competency test staff. The in-home competency evaluation tool is completed on orientation and as part of the performance appraisal process.
7. Nurses, therapists, and social workers are competency tested annually.
8. Speech pathologists are competency tested by the contractor on an annual basis.
9. Advanced practice nurses (staff and contract) possess a master's degree in an area of clinical practice and a clinical specialist certification or certification/registration as a nurse practitioner. Competencies are generally cognitive in nature and are maintained through educational activities and, when indicated, skills demonstration.
10. Home health aides: Refer to Policy 1:27, Home Health Aide/Homemaker Services,

2. Verification validates the paper document.
3. The form enables a clinical educator or clinical supervisor to ascertain areas of weakness and ensure that staff or contractors gain these skills.
4. The discipline specific orientation contain basic competencies which must be validated.
5. Competency testing may be done in a lab setting or in a patient's home.

6. The in-home competency evaluation tool contains standards that the department deems necessary for the safe provision of care. The tool allows the supervisor to assess the maintenance of staff's skills on an annual basis.
7. The goal is to improve the competency of staff by an ongoing assessment of educational needs.
8. Speech pathologists are competency tested by their employer. In addition, the contractor requires the therapist to obtain a Certificate of Clinical Competence.
9. Preparation at the master's level as a clinical nurse specialist or nurse practitioner presumes competence. Certification requires ongoing education, publication, and/or presentations in a specialty area.

and Policy, 1:28, Home Health Aide Training, Certification, and Competency Evaluation Program.
11. Volunteers: Refer to Policy 1:72, Volunteer Services.
12. The dietitian is registered by the Commission on Dietetic Registration, the credentialing agency for the American Dietetic Association, and is certified by the National Certification Board for Diabetic Education. Competencies are generally cognitive in nature and are maintained through educational activities.

12. In addition to successful completion of a registration exam, registered dietitians must complete 75 hours of continuing education every five years. A Certified Diabetic Educator must complete 1,000 hours of diabetic patient education, sit for an exam every five years, meet professional education requirements in effect at the time of recertification, and submit proof of current unrestricted U.S. license/registration.

13. Hospice team members, medical director, chaplin, volunteers, and dietitians are competency tested through educational activities and/or performance evaluations and, when indicated, skills demonstration.

13. Clinical educator and hospice coordinator maintain responsibility for hospice competency testing.

14. Select contractor organizations will be required to show evidence of competency testing. In addition, the department reserves the right to competency test through orientation, educational activities, and/or skills demonstration.

14. Select contracts will require evidence of competency testing. The department will ascertain if additional competencies are required.

15. The director of quality improvement, in conjunction with the clinical educator, collects, aggregates, and analyzes data on staff competency to ascertain learning needs.

15. The department uses a collaborative approach to analyze staff competency needs. Information is collected from quality indicators, staff education meetings, test scores, and supervisors' meetings and reported to supervisory and administrative staff.

Reference: The Maryland Healthcare Education Institute, "Developing a Comprehensive Competency Program" (Program Material). Presented by Camilla Rogers, MSN.

Origin Date: _____
Revised Date: _____
Approved Date: _____
Originator: _____
Distribution: _____

1:14
CONFLICT OF INTEREST

PURPOSE:

To request the disclosure of potential conflicts of interest so that appropriate action may be taken to ensure that such conflict does not inappropriately influence decision making

RESPONSIBLE PERSONNEL:

All staff

OBJECTIVES:

- To conduct patient care and other business operations in an ethical manner consistent with the hospital and home care department's mission
- To express commitment to the protection and dignity of the rights of all patients
- To ensure that all employees recognize the importance of their work responsibilities and understand the need to communicate any outside employment activities
- To avoid personal gain or advantage to the individual
- To avoid an adverse effect of the employee's interest
- To avoid improper gain or advantage to a third-party

POLICY:

Any employee engaged in outside employment/consultation activity will observe the highest standards of professional ethics and avoid any activity that is not in the best interest of the hospital or home care department.

PROCEDURE:

1. Newly hired employees will report all outside employment/consultation activity on their employment application.
2. It is the responsibility of all regular full-time and part-time employees to inform their department management of any outside employment/consultation activity in a timely manner.
3. *Guidelines:* Outside employment should not:
   a. Have an adverse effect on performance, for example:
      - Employees' performance declines because of fatigue
      - Inability to work overtime
      - Working for outside interests on hospital time
      - Creating a scheduling conflict and/or being absent an abnormal amount of time due to such conflict
   b. Create a conflict of interest situation, for example, an employee working
      - for another company that provides goods or services to the hospital
      - as a consultant for a company where he or she could divulge confidential hospital information
      - for a supplier where there is a possibility of influencing purchases of hospital services
4. Failure to comply with this policy may subject the employee to disciplinary action as outlined in personnel policy.

5. The decision about the existence of a conflict of interest is the responsibility of the executive director or designee, in consultation with the human resource department.

Origin Date: _____
Revised Date: _____
Approved Date: _____
Originator: _____
Distribution: _____

**1:15
CORE SERVICES**

PHYSICIAN

- The hospice physician who serves as the medical director of the interdisciplinary group is a licensed physician who, on the basis of training, experience, and interest, is knowledgeable about hospice care. The physician is an advisor to the hospice team in areas of pain and symptom control and in other elements of medical management. The hospice physician complements the patient's primary physician in providing a medical resource to the team to promote optimal patient care. The hospice physician shall, in addition to assisting with the palliation and management of the terminal illness, meet the general medical needs of the hospice patients to the extent that these needs are not met by the attending physician.

NURSING SERVICES

- Nursing is provided by primary nurses who have received additional education in hospice care. Hospice cases are assigned to the hospice nurses by either the coordinator or the clinical supervisor. Substantially all nursing services are provided directly by the hospice.
- Nurses are assigned to hospice patients for the duration of their care needs to ensure continuity of care. If a substitute nurse is needed for staff coverage, he or she will follow the interdisciplinary group plan of care under the guidance of the hospice coordinator.
- Nurses who are not hospice trained may co-carry a hospice patient in their area with a hospice primary nurse. Hospice nursing activities are under the guidance of the hospice coordinator. Nursing services are available on a visit basis according to the need. Frequency of visits will be based on assessment of patients' needs.
- Nursing services include evaluation of the patient with appropriate notification to the interdisciplinary group of changes in the patient's condition, implementation of changes in the plan of treatment, and instruction and supervision of various aspects of the patient's care to all professional or paraprofessional personnel involved with the patient in the home setting.

MEDICAL SOCIAL SERVICES

- Medical social services are provided by a qualified social worker under the direction of the physician as evidenced in the plan of care. The social worker is available to provide counseling services to the hospice patients and their families or others providing care in the home. The social worker assists in facilitation of communication for patients and families and assists in referrals to other resources as needed for optimal patient care.

COUNSELING SERVICES

- *Pastoral Counseling:* Pastoral counseling services are provided by an ordained minister, who may serve as liaison with the patient's own clergy or provide direct spiritual support to the patient and family as indicated by patient/family needs and requests.
- *Nutrition Counseling:* Nutrition and diet counseling is available and will be provided by a registered dietitian. The registered dietitian, under the guidance of the hospice interdisciplinary group, shall provide assessment of hospice patients' nutrition needs and guidance of appropriate nutrition therapy.
- *Psychiatric Counseling:* Psychiatric counseling is provided by a master's prepared nurse specialist in psychiatric or mental health nursing. The psychiatric nurse clinician will be available to hospice patients and families who are experiencing complex emotional and/or psychiatric problems. The psychiatric nurse clinician will be referred to patients at the direction of the interdisciplinary group.
- *Bereavement Counseling:* Refer to Bereavement Program Policy, 1:08.

OTHER SERVICES

- *Physical Therapy, Occupational Therapy, Speech Pathology:* These three services are available to hospice patients under the direction of the interdisciplinary group as needed to provide symptom control or to enable the patient to maximize activities of daily living and basic functional skills.
- *Home Health Aides/Homemakers:* Qualified home health aides and homemakers are available to provide personal care services and household services to maintain a safe and sanitary environment for the patient. The home health aide functions under the supervision and direction of the primary hospice nurse and follows the plan of care established by the nurse. The home health aide will be supervised by the primary hospice nurse at least every two weeks.
- *Medical Supplies:* For Medicare hospice benefit patients, medical supplies and appliances, including drugs and biologicals, are provided as needed for palliation of symptoms and management of their terminal illness and related conditions. Medical supplies and appliances are provided as outlined in the patient's hospice benefit for those patients who elect the benefit. For those patients who do not specifically have coverage by third-party payers, the home care hospice program will attempt to secure services for optimal patient care.
- *Inpatient Care for Symptom Control:*
  - For Medicare hospice benefit patients, inpatient care for pain control and symptom management will be provided under the direction of the interdisciplinary group plan of care at Abington Memorial Hospital. Abington Memorial Hospital has designated hospice beds to enhance the quality of acute inpatient care. The focus of the inpatient care is acute care symptom management for short periods of time. An inpatient hospice case manager position has been established to coordinate acute care, establish the plan of care in collaboration with the IDG, and promote continuity.

- For other (not hospice benefit) hospice patients requiring short-term hospital admissions, the interdisciplinary group will maintain close communications with the inpatient setting to promote continuity of care.
- *Inpatient Care for Respite:*
  - Inpatient care for respite will be provided for hospice benefit patients at contract facilities. Skilled nursing facility respite care is furnished under the direction of the interdisciplinary group plan of care to relieve the individual's family or other persons providing care in the home.
  - Respite care may be provided only on an occasional basis. The duration of respite stay is determined by the individual's insurance plan. Medicare hospice benefit respite stay is no longer than five consecutive days. During the inpatient respite stay, the hospice nurse or designee will make contact daily to assess the patient, review the plan of care, and establish continuity (if necessary). Contact with the facility will be made on admission to transfer the plan of treatment.
  - For those patients who do not elect their hospice benefit, the home care department will attempt to secure optimal respite care as available for patient/family care.

Origin Date: _____
Revised Date: _____
Approved Date: _____
Originator: _____
Distribution: _____

1:16
DEATH PRONOUNCEMENT BY REGISTERED NURSES

PURPOSE:

To provide a description of the scope of practice for registered nurses who provide home health and hospice care

RESPONSIBLE PERSONNEL:

Registered nurses

OBJECTIVES:

- To provide quality of care throughout the life cycle, including the time of death
- To determine the absence of vital signs for patients who are currently receiving home health and hospice care
- To facilitate the release of the body of the deceased to a funeral director after notice has been given to the attending physician and to a family member

POLICY:

Professional nurses may pronounce death and release the body of the deceased as specified in Pennsylvania Act 46 (Section 507, Death and Fetal Death Registration: Pronouncement of Death by a Professional Nurse), signed into law by Governor Casey December 20, 1991 and effective February 19, 1992.
- Professional nurses licensed under the act of May 22, 1951 (P.L. 317, No. 69) known as the "The Professional Nursing Law," as amended, who are involved in direct care of a patient shall have the authority to pronounce death as determined under the act of

December 17, 1982 (P.L. 1401, No. 323), known as the "Uniform Determination of Death Act," in the case of death from natural causes of a patient who is under the care of a physician when the physician is unable to be present within reasonable period of time to certify the cause of death. For this policy "who are involved in direct care" means patients under the direct care of a professional nurse employed by this agency.

- Only an individual who has sustained either of the following is dead:
  - irreversible cessation of circulatory and respiratory functions
  - irreversible cessation of all functions of the entire brain including the brain stem

  A determination of death must be made in accordance with accepted medical standards (Uniform Determination of Death Act).
- Professional nurses shall have the authority to release the body of the deceased to a funeral director after notice has been given to the attending physician, when the deceased has an attending physician, and to a family member.
- If circumstances surrounding the nature of death are not anticipated and require a coroner's investigation, the professional nurse shall notify the county coroner, and the release to the funeral home shall be the responsibility of the coroner.
- The pronouncement of death by professional nurses shall be in accordance with the Uniform Determination of Death Act, which in no way authorizes a nurse to determine the cause of death. The responsibility for determining the cause of death remains with the physician or coroner.
- Responsibility and liability:
  - Professional nurses and employing agencies of professional nurses acting in good faith and in compliance with the guidelines established by Act 46 and the State Board of Nursing shall be immune from liability claims by reason of pronouncing death.
  - Nothing contained in this Act shall be deemed to impose any obligation upon a professional nurse to carry out the function authorized by this Act.
  - Nothing in this Act is intended to relieve a professional nurse of any civil or criminal liability that might otherwise be incurred for failing to follow the rules and regulations of the State Board of Nursing.
  - Nothing in this Act shall preempt the requirements of the provision of 20 Pennsylvania CS CH86 (relating to anatomical gifts).

PROCEDURE:

Action	Rationale
1. Administrator will order Commonwealth of Pennsylvania Certificate of Death forms.	1. The official document will be available in home health/hospice agency for registered nurses.
2. The nurse will determine the presence or absence of vital signs.	2. The nurse identifies and discriminates between physical signs essential to life.
3. The nurse will notify the attending physician. When the physician is contacted but is not available to sign certificate, the nurse will leave death certificate with the family. The funeral director will ensure that the physician completes and signs certificate.	3. The nurse will comply with the law.

4. The nurse will notify a family member.
5. The nurse will complete the following selected portions of the Certificate of Death, Commonwealth of Pennsylvania, Vital Statistics Form H105.143 (other sections of the form will be completed by the funeral director and physician):
   - Block 1— Name of deceased
   - Block 4—Date of death
   - Block 8a—Check the box "Other" and specify: Home
   - Block 23a—Signature of registered nurse
   - Block 23b—RN license number
   - Block 23c—Date signed
   - Block 24—Time of death
   - Block 25—Date pronounced dead
   - Block 26—Was case referred to medical examiner/coroner*
6. The nurse will notify the funeral director and provide the name of physician.
7. The nurse will disclose HIV-related information to the funeral director responsible for the acceptance and preparation of the deceased patient.
8. The nurse will complete documentation in clinical record.
9. The nurse provides emotional support to family members.

4. The nurse will comply with the law.
5. The nurse will comply with the law.

6. The nurse will initiate completion of the certificate of death and facilitate removal of the body of the deceased.
7. The nurse provides required information and compliance with Pennsylvania law (Act 148, Confidentiality of HIV-Related Information Act of 1990).
8. The nurse will meet professional and agency standards.
9. The nurse provides quality care.

To order Certificates of Death, place order in writing to:
   Division of Vital Statistics
   P.O. Box 1528
   New Castle, PA 16103
Allow two weeks for processing.

Origin Date: _____
Revised Date: _____
Approved Date: _____
Originator: _____
Distribution: _____

---

*Note: Pennsylvania law (Act 1990-152) requires that all cases where the body is to be cremated, buried at sea, or otherwise disposed of, so as to be thereafter unavailable to examination, must be reported to the coroner of the county. Effective in 1991, all deaths in which remains are to be cremated must be referred to the coroner's office having jurisdiction over the death.

On May 28, 1992, the Montgomery County Commissioner approved a motion that a permit fee shall be charged to all funeral directors requesting permission to cremate a body (Title 16 of County Code PS1237, subsection A). This mandates that the coroner investigate the facts and circumstances concerning deaths happening within the county whereby the deceased's body would be disposed of in such a manner as to thereafter make it unavailable for any future examination.

1:17
DISCHARGE POLICIES

REQUIREMENTS FOR DISCHARGE

A. Discharge will be approved when:
   1. Patient/family refuse service and physician is notified.
   2. Patient's residence is changed to a geographic area not serviced by the hospice.
   3. Patient requests a transfer to another hospice.
   4. Patient elects to revoke the hospice benefit.
   5. Physician's orders are not renewed in accordance with established policy.
   6. Physician refuses to certify the patient as terminally ill.
   7. Patient/family refuse to cooperate in achievement of the established objectives.
   8. The basic facilities conducive to a health environment become inadequate.
   9. Patient expires. Bereavement services will continue following a patient's death.
   10. Patient's condition improves and he or she is no longer considered terminally ill.
B. Upon termination of service, a discharge summary, including the date and reason for discharge, shall be entered on the patient's record.
C. If discharge occurs prior to the patient's death, home care policy regarding discharge and transfer of patients is followed.

PLEASE NOTE:

If the patient is discharged from AMH Home Care Hospice, he or she may be eligible for skilled intermittent services offered by AMH Home Care.

Origin Date: _____
Revised Date: _____
Approved Date: _____
Originator: _____
Distribution: _____

1:18
DISPOSAL OF CONTROLLED DRUGS

- When controlled drugs are no longer needed by the patient in the home, the hospice shall instruct the patient's caregiver in proper disposal.
- The patient's family shall be instructed to flush the remaining controlled drugs down the toilet. If the hospice team member destroys the drugs at the family's request, a family member should be present. The hospice team member shall document the instructions regarding the disposal of drugs and outcomes in the clinical record.
- Families may also be instructed to contact the physician regarding disposition of narcotics.
- Contract pharmacists will be notified of hospice benefit patients' death to prevent further refill of controlled pharmaceuticals.

Origin Date: _____
Revised Date: _____
Approved Date: _____
Originator: _____
Distribution: _____

1:19
DISPOSAL OF USED SYRINGES

PURPOSE:

To establish and carry out a procedure to dispose of used syringes to protect against unauthorized use or unacceptable contamination

RESPONSIBLE PERSONNEL:

Director of professional services, professional nursing staff

OBJECTIVES:

To establish a procedure to dispose of all used syringes that conforms with safety guidelines for disposal of contaminated material and to protect against unauthorized use

POLICY:

Syringes used by the nurse shall be disposed of in a manner that is safe for the patient, the caregiver, and the general public.

PROCEDURE:

Action	Rationale
1. Nurses return all syringes used in the care of patients in a labeled red sharps container to the home care office. The sharps container is placed in a red biohazard bag for transport.	1. Syringes should be disposed of in a safe manner.
2. Periodically, the designated support staff arrange with the contractor for disposal. Upon arrival at the office, the bagged sharps container is placed in a large red biohazard container where it is held until disposal.	2. An agency is required to provide for safe disposal of used syringes.
3. The contracted medical waste company transports the waste and incinerates it as per state laws.	3. Incineration is a safe method of syringe disposal.
4. A copy of the manifest is kept in Abington Properties Corporation.	4. The manifest meets Pennsylvania Department of Environmental Resources (DER) regulations.

Origin Date: _____
Revised Date: _____
Approved Date: _____
Originator: _____
Distribution: _____

1:20
DO NOT RESUSCITATE

PURPOSE:
- To establish policy for do not resuscitate (DNR) procedures in the provision of care to hospice patients
- To ensure that written instructions are in place in the event of a life-threatening situation for a hospice patient

RESPONSIBLE PERSONNEL:
Visiting staff, hospice interdisciplinary group, patient's attending physician

OBJECTIVES:
- To establish the hospice's policy concerning DNR for hospice patients
- To establish guidelines for agency personnel in the discussion and documentation of DNR orders for hospice patients
- To secure DNR orders on hospice patients in a timely fashion with the interdisciplinary plan of care

POLICY:
- The philosophy of hospice includes the concept that hospice care neither prolongs life nor hastens death.
- In the event of a hospice patient's cardiac or respiratory arrest, cardiopulmonary resuscitation measures will not be initiated.

PROCEDURE:

Action	Rationale
1. DNR status will be discussed with the patient/family and hospice team during admitting home visits for hospice.	1. Hospice recognizes the need for patients to maintain control over their own care and to let others (caregiver) know their wishes regarding resuscitation.
2. The DNR status will be included in the patient's authorization/informed consent form.	2. The patient's wishes regarding resuscitation should be clearly reflected in the chart.
3. The patient/family decision regarding DNR is periodically reassessed and documented in progress notes.	3. The patient/family decision should clearly reflect the current patient condition. Staff should recognize that informed consent is a continuing process with ongoing

4. A physician's order is obtained regarding the patient/family preference for resuscitation and is included in the interdisciplinary plan of care.
5. All DNR decisions are communicated to persons involved in providing hospice care, including inpatient facilities.
6. Changes and amendments to the DNR orders are documented by the team and physician.

4. The physician has a responsibility to discuss the implications of DNR and to respect the patient's decisions regarding DNR.
5. Communications should be clear regarding DNR in the event of a life-threatening situation.
6. Communications regarding DNR should be clear.

Origin Date: _____
Revised Date: _____
Approved Date: _____
Originator: _____
Distribution: _____

1:21
ELIGIBILITY REQUIREMENTS FOR MEDICARE HOSPICE BENEFIT

To elect hospice care under Medicare, an individual must be
- entitled to Part A of Medicare and
- certified as being terminally ill by both the hospice medical director and the patient's attending physician

ELECTION OF HOSPICE CARE:

- For patients who are eligible for Medicare hospice benefits:
  - The patient or representative may file an election statement with the Abington Memorial Hospital Home Care Hospice Program. The election statement will designate the first effective date of hospice care and subsequent election periods.
  - The duration of the election of hospice care shall continue through the initial period and through the subsequent election periods without a break in care as long as the individual remains in the care of AMHHC Hospice and does not revoke the election under the provisions of COP 418.28.
  - The patient or representative shall receive a full explanation of the palliative nature of hospice from the admitting hospice nurse or social worker, and this will be described on the election statement.
  - The election statement includes identification of the AMHHC Hospice Program as the hospice provider and the acknowledgment that certain Medicare services are waived by the election.
  - For patients who are not eligible for or do not elect the Medicare hospice benefit, the individual or representative will receive an explanation of hospice services available and sign the AMHHC Hospice Authorization and Release Form.

REVOKING ELECTION OF HOSPICE CARE:

- An individual or representative may revoke the individual's election of hospice care at any time during an election period. To revoke the election of hospice care, the individual

or representative must file a statement with the hospice that includes the effective date of revocation and the understanding of the individual or representative that the remainder of the current benefit period for hospice is forfeited but that the individual may at any future time elect other election periods that he or she may be eligible to receive.
- Patients who revoke hospice care will be informed that, if eligible, they may resume hospice care with the agency in the future. Patients' attending physicians will also be informed if patients revoke hospice care.

Origin Date: _____
Revised Date: _____
Approved Date: _____
Originator: _____
Distribution: _____

1:22
EMERGENCY PHONE NUMBERS

(List important contact people and their phone numbers.)

PROCEDURE:

1. Call the hospice coordinator with hospice patient problems after office hours.
2. Call clinical supervisors if hospice coordinator does not answer.

Origin Date: _____
Revised Date: _____
Approved Date: _____
Originator: _____
Distribution: _____

1:23
EMERGENCY PREPAREDNESS PLAN

PURPOSE:

To establish a plan that will provide continuing care and support appropriate to the provision of care in the event of an emergency

RESPONSIBLE PERSONNEL:

All staff

OBJECTIVES:

- To provide guidance and direction to staff during a time of crisis
- To identify service priorities
- To identify community resources available to the department during a crisis

POLICY:

The organization has an established written plan known by all staff for providing continuing care and support to all patients to the extent possible based on the patient's needs in the event of an emergency.

DEFINITION:

A disaster is a natural or manmade event that significantly disrupts the environment, such as damage to the agency's building, hurricanes, snowstorms, or thunderstorms. Disasters also include events that disrupt services, such as loss of utilities (power, telephone), or emergencies in the surrounding community, such as industrial accidents. (*Note:* Definition revised to describe disasters specific to this region.)

PROCEDURE:

Action	Rationale
1. The mechanism used to contact staff in an emergency is a phone tree, which is initiated by the executive director and/or the director of professional services. Each supervisor is expected to contact his or her respective staff with specific instructions.	1. Communication with staff is a priority during an emergency situation.
2. In the event that the office phone system is disrupted and we lose call forwarding to the answering service, calls are directed to the hospital operator. On-call nurses are directed to contact the hospital operator for messages. The operators may also contact home care administrative/supervisory staff.	2. The hospital phone system provides a backup for the home care system. The director of communications has established home care as a priority to reactivate call forwarding when the phone system becomes operational.
3. In the event that regional communication is disrupted, administrative and supervisory staff will attempt to contact staff through their personal beepers and cellular phones. In addition, when deemed appropriate, information will be communicated to staff via the public broadcasting system (i.e., radio).	3. Supervisors and administrative staff keep a list of personal cellular phone and beeper numbers.
4. In the event of a community or weather-related crisis, staff are expected to report to work. During periods of severe weather, staff are instructed to take patient demographic and clinical data to their homes. Demographic and clinical information may be accessed in the Clinical Link Computer System by laptop computer. If a weather emergency occurs, staff may be asked to evaluate and prioritize from their homes.	4. Every effort is made to meet the urgent needs of patients during inclement weather. Computerization of the patient record allows for immediate access of patient information.

5. Cases are evaluated and prioritized by the administrative, supervisory, and clinical staff.
6. In the event that visits cannot be made, patients/families are instructed to provide the care themselves. Staff provide individualized phone instruction to the patient or family, guiding them on the specific treatment or procedure.
7. Clients with emergency needs that the staff cannot meet will be referred to hospital emergency departments, acute care facilities, nursing homes, neighboring home health agencies, or other available community resources are contacted, such as
   - family physician
   - hospital (emergency departments)
   - local police
   - ambulance service (local ambulance companies)
8. In the event that the hospital implements the disaster plan, staff will be available to make home visits to discharged patients.
9. The hospital nurse case managers will report to their respective units to facilitate rapid discharge of patients.
10. The home care department will work in conjunction with the department of nursing as stipulated in the nursing department's disaster plan.
11. In the event of a fire emergency, staff will follow the plan as posted.
12. If destruction of the building occurs, arrangements will be made for operations to be conducted out of the hospital. The information services department will retrieve the computer backup disks, which are stored off-site. Patient clinical and demographic information will be restored for distribution to staff. The department's policy and procedure manual is copied on disk and stored off-site.
13. The emergency preparedness plan is evaluated.

5. Patients categorized as highest priority receive service first.
6. Patients and families are usually able to rise to the emergency if they are given individualized/personal guidance over the phone.
7. Patients are referred to an appropriate source to meet needs unable to be provided by home care staff. No patient is left without help.
8. The hospital disaster plan calls for immediate discharge of stable patients to allow for rapid influx of the sick and injured. Hospital admission may be averted with home care follow-up.
9. The hospital nurse case managers will facilitate rapid discharge, which will increase the number of beds available to the sick and injured.
10. Coordination of services with the nursing department will allow for optimum utilization of staff.
11. Every effort is made to protect safety of staff in the event of a fire.
12. All computer information (clinical, statistical, billing) is copied on disk daily and stored off-site.
13. Evaluation compliance with Joint Commission standards.

Origin Date: _____
Revised Date: _____
Approved Date: _____
Originator: _____
Distribution: _____

1:24
EXPOSURE CONTROL PLAN

POLICY:

It is the policy of Abington Memorial Hospital Home Care Department to prevent the transmission of bloodborne pathogens by minimizing the exposure of personnel in all departments to blood and body fluids of all patients. The methods to be employed in reducing exposure of personnel are outlined in this plan. The components in the exposure control plan and referenced policies are designed to comply with Part 1910, Section 1910.1030 of Title 29 of the Code of Federal Regulations.

EXPOSURE DETERMINATION AND CLASSIFICATION

A. Each employee and volunteer job description will be reviewed and classified according to the potential for exposure to blood or other potentially infectious materials.
   1. Potentially infectious materials other than blood are
      a. semen, vaginal secretions, cerebrospinal fluid, synovial fluid, pleural fluid, peritoneal fluid, pericardial fluid, amniotic fluid, saliva in dental procedures, any body fluid that visibly contains blood, and all body fluids where it is difficult to differentiate between body fluids
      b. any unfixed tissue or organ other than intact skin
   2. Assignment of classification will be made without regard to the use of barriers and other personal protective equipment.
B. Classifications of exposure are as follows:
   1. *Exposed Employees:* Employees and volunteers in this classification have reasonably anticipated skin, eye, mucous membrane, or parenteral contact with blood or other potentially infectious materials that may result from the performance of assigned duties. For the purposes of this policy, "employees" will refer to both employees and volunteers.
   2. *Nonexposed Employees:* Employees in this classification have no reasonably anticipated skin, eye, mucous membrane, or parenteral contact with blood or other potentially infectious materials that may result from the performance of their duties.
C. Job titles classified as exposed include clinical supervisors, nurse practitioners, home care nurses, home health aide patient care attendants, and home clinical nurse specialists.

METHODS OF COMPLIANCE

Universal Blood and Body Fluid Precautions

A. Universal precautions shall be observed to prevent contact with blood and other potentially infectious materials.

B. The policy of universal blood and body fluid precautions has been in effect since December 1987. See Infection Control: Universal Blood and Body Fluid Precautions (1:33) for specifics.

Engineering and Work Practice Controls

A. Engineering and work practice controls shall be used to eliminate or minimize employee exposure.
   1. Where occupational exposure remains after institution of these controls, personal protective equipment shall also be used.
   2. The professional advisory committee shall review work practice controls on an annual basis. This is done by an extensive review of policy and procedures, including a review of trends in employee exposures.
B. See Infection Control: Universal Blood and Body Fluid Precautions (1:33), for specifics regarding engineering and work practice controls such as use of personal protective equipment, handling and disposal of contaminated sharps, handling of specimens, and use of warning labels and signs.
C. Managers and supervisors shall ensure the compliance of employees with the requirements of universal blood and body fluid precautions.

Handwashing Requirements

A. Employees shall wash hands and any other potentially contaminated skin area with soap and water immediately or as soon as feasible after removing gloves.
B. Handwashing facilities are generally available in most homes. Antiseptic towelettes or alcohol-based handwashing solutions may be used as a temporary substitute for handwashing. Hands shall be washed with soap and water as soon as feasible.
C. See infection control policy for other handwashing specifics.

Personal Protective Equipment

A. See universal blood and body fluid precautions policy for specifics regarding the use and provision of personal protective equipment.
B. Supervisors shall ensure that employees use appropriate personal protective equipment. If an employee declines to use personal protective equipment based on a judgment that use of protective equipment would prevent delivery of care or would pose an increased hazard, the circumstances shall be investigated. The investigation must be documented on an Employee Conference Form, including a determination of whether changes can be instituted to prevent such occurrences. The completed Employee Conference Form will be forwarded to the personnel department.
C. Housekeeping: See infection control policy for specifics regarding housekeeping requirements and management of spills.

HEPATITIS B VACCINATION

A. The hepatitis B vaccine is available at no cost to all employees whose jobs are classified as exposed. The vaccine is administered by the staff of employee/student health under the supervision of the physician director.

B. Hepatitis B vaccine will be made available to all employees whose jobs are classified as exposed after the employees have received training and within 10 working days of initial assignment.
C. Exposed employees who decline hepatitis B vaccination shall sign a statement of declination.
D. For exposed employees who decline hepatitis B vaccination but later—while still employed in an exposed job classification—elect to accept vaccination, the vaccination will be provided at no cost.

POSTEXPOSURE EVALUATION AND FOLLOW-UP

A. Following significant exposures, medical evaluation and treatment, including the hepatitis B vaccine, appropriate testing, and prophylaxis, are available without cost to all employees.
   1. Following significant exposures, immediate evaluation, including route of exposure, circumstances of exposure, and identification of source individual, is conducted by a registered professional nurse as specified in infection control policy. After initial evaluation, employees are evaluated and treated in the emergency/trauma center or employee student health.
   2. Employees will be offered HIV and HBV antibody testing as part of postexposure evaluation. If an employee consents to blood collection but declines HIV testing at the time of the evaluation, the blood specimen will be saved in the lab for 90 days. If the employee elects to have HIV and/or HBV antibody testing within the 90 day period, such testing will be performed.
B. Information to be provided to employee/student health includes the following:
   1. A copy of the Occupational Safety and Health Administration Rule 1910.1030, Occupational Exposure to Bloodborne Pathogens, will be maintained in employee/student health for reference.
   2. The AMH Employee Accident and Illness Report and the AMH Needlestick—Blood/Body Fluid Exposure Form are to be completed at the time of the exposure incident and presented to employee/student health at the time of evaluation. These forms are to include
      - a description of the exposure incident including route(s) of exposure and surrounding circumstances
      - results of source individual's blood testing if available
   3. A history of vaccination status will be maintained in employee/student health.
C. Employee/student health will provide the employee with a copy of the evaluating physician's written opinion within 15 days of the completion of the evaluation. The written opinion will include
   1. whether the hepatitis B vaccination is indicated for the employee and whether the employee has received such vaccination
   2. documentation that the employee has been informed of the results of the evaluation
   3. documentation that the employee has been told about any medical conditions resulting from exposure to blood or other potentially infectious materials that require further evaluation or treatment
   4. other findings or diagnoses shall remain confidential and not be included in the written report
D. Medical recordkeeping:

1. Employee/student health shall establish and maintain an accurate record for each employee with occupational exposure, including volunteers with exposure. Records shall include
   - name and Social Security number of employee
   - copy of employee's hepatitis B vaccination status including the dates of administration and/or
     - antibody testing that demonstrates immunity
     - documentation that the employee has received the vaccination previously
     - copies of documentation required for postexposure evaluation and follow-up, including a copy of written opinion provided to the employee
2. Records are to be kept confidential and shall not be disclosed or reported without the employee's express written consent to any person within or outside the workplace except as required by law.
3. Records shall be maintained for the duration of employment plus 30 years.

COMMUNICATION OF HAZARDS TO EMPLOYEES

A. Labels and signs: See infection control policy for specifics regarding appropriate use of biohazard labels and other identification of infectious materials.
B. Information and training:
   1. All employees with occupational exposure must receive training
      - at the time of initial assignment to tasks involving potential occupational exposure
      - at least annually thereafter
      - as specified in section (g)(2) of Occupational Safety and Health Administration Rule 1910.1030, Occupational Exposure to Bloodborne Pathogens
   2. Copies of annual training records will be submitted to the department of epidemiology. Training records shall be maintained for three years from the date on which the training occurred. Training records shall include the following:
      - date(s) of training sessions
      - contents or summary of sessions
      - names and qualifications of persons conducting training
      - names and job titles of persons attending

EFFECTIVE DATES

A. The home care department's exposure control plan will be distributed to the epidemiology department for review and approval. The plan will be distributed to exposed employees. The requirements of the plan will become effective as follows:
   1. Information, training, and recordkeeping requirements become effective June 4, 1992.
   2. Engineering and work practice controls, personal protective equipment, housekeeping, hepatitis B vaccination and postexposure evaluation and follow-up, and labels and signs requirements become effective July 6, 1992.
   3. The exposure control plan will be reviewed and revised as needed at least annually. The professional advisory committee will approve all reviews and revisions of the plan.

Origin Date: _____
Revised Date: _____
Approved Date: _____
Originator: _____
Distribution: _____

1:25
GOVERNING BODY

The hospice program, as a program of the Abington Memorial Hospital Home Care Department, is governed by the board of trustees of the hospital. The governing body assumes full responsibility for determining, implementing, and monitoring policies governing the hospice's total operation, designating an individual responsible for the day-to-day management of the program, and ensuring compliance with accepted standards of practice.

PROCESS FOR REPORTING HOME CARE AND HOSPICE PROGRAM INFORMATION

- The executive director reports to the executive vice president through regularly scheduled meetings (usually every two weeks).
- The executive vice president reports issues and concerns to the board of trustees at its scheduled meetings. If there is no problem, there is no report.
- The formal method for reporting to the board of trustees is through the performance improvement (PI) committee. This occurs on a quarterly basis. The reports of all departments are shared with the PI committee. The board of trustees is represented on the PI committee. Department directors are invited to attend the committee meeting on an annual basis to present the report.

Origin Date: _____
Revised Date: _____
Approved Date: _____
Originator: _____
Distribution: _____

1:26
HOME CARE SERVICES

- The hospice program is part of the home care program of Abington Memorial Hospital's Home Care (AMHHC) Department and, as such, follows the general policies and procedures of the AMHHC.
- Services are available to hospice patients 24 hours a day, seven days a week, and are covered after hours by the nurse on call according to the home care answering service policy. Hospice patients who have an IV are also covered by the IV on-call nurse.
- Care for patients who are receiving hospice benefit services will be managed by the hospice interdisciplinary group in coordination with the attending physician. As per

contracts with AMHHC Hospice Program, the patient's acute care will be managed at Abington Memorial Hospital, and respite care will be provided at contracted facilities. Pharmaceuticals will be obtained from contracted pharmacies and durable medical equipment and supplies from contracted medical equipment companies. Laboratory and radiology treatment will be secured at the direction of the hospice from Abington Memorial Hospital. Emergency treatment for illnesses/injuries not related to the terminal illness will be managed by the patient's attending physician or at the hospital of his or her choice.

- For laboratory, radiology, and emergency treatment, the nonbenefit patient is referred to the hospital of the attending physician's choice.
- Treatment modalities such as intravenous procedures, chemotherapy, parenteral feedings, and injections will be obtained from infusion service as per contract. These treatments are covered by the professional services policies and procedures of the home care department. The purpose of these therapeutic modalities for hospice patients is palliation rather than cure.
- The administration of investigational drugs is covered by the professional service policies of AMHHC.
- Documentation of medications, side effects, and potential interactions are found in the AMHHC clinical record. The hospice team has access to resources in pharmacology, including the medical director, the professional advisory board, the hospice nurse coordinator, and various literature.
- The actions taken by the hospice team members present at the patient's death or following the patient's death are according to the professional service policies of the home care department.
- The disposal of narcotic medications is according to the home care department professional service policies.

Origin Date: _____
Revised Date: _____
Approved Date: _____
Originator: _____
Distribution: _____

1:27
HOME HEALTH AIDE/HOMEMAKER SERVICES

PURPOSE:

To provide a description of the scope of practice of home health aide/homemaker services in the home care/hospice program

RESPONSIBLE PERSONNEL:

Director of professional services, home health aides, professional nurses, therapists

OBJECTIVES:

- To provide personal care and support to ill and disabled persons in the home for the achievement of a continuity in basic health care

- To assist in basic therapeutic services to patients under the direction and supervision of physical and occupational therapists

POLICY:

- Qualified home health aides and homemakers work as members of the home care/hospice team under the direction and guidance of a physician and a professional nurse or therapist.
- The assignment is made in accordance with a plan of care prescribed by the physician and established by the nurse. A visit schedule and appropriate written instructions with the plans of care are made available under the supervision of a registered nurse or therapist. The home health aide/homemaker is responsible for the completion of all necessary home health aide records.
- Services provided are to be within the scope and limitations set forth in the plan of care and may not be altered in type, scope, or duration by the aide, the patient, the family, or the contracting agency.
- Home health aides provide personal care and assist with basic therapeutic services to persons in their homes who are ill or disabled. Homemakers provide minimal assistance with physical care, concentrating their efforts on other household activities. These services are initiated when the following criteria are met:
  - The patient is currently admitted to the agency's services.
  - There is a physician's plan of care that orders the services.
  - A professional nurse has assessed the patient's needs and determined that home health aide/homemaker services are needed.
  - The professional nurse has developed a plan of care.
  - The nurse has oriented the home health aide or homemaker to the patient care situation and the plan of care.
  - The nurse is providing supportive supervision and teaching to the home health aide/homemaker as needed, but at least every two weeks.
  - The nurse is available to provide prompt guidance and assistance when indicated.

PROCEDURE:

Action	Rationale
1. Home health aide services are provided by a qualified home health aide in accordance with a plan of care prescribed by a physician and the written visit schedule and written instructions from the supervising nurse or therapist. The home health aide carries out the following functions: • Provides simple patient care, including bath, back massage, application of lotion for lubrication of the skin, oral hygiene, nail care, shampoo, positioning of bed patient, patient transferred to and from bed or chair, feed-	1. These measures constitute the scope of home health aide practice in a home care setting and comply with Medicare Conditions of Participation.

ing patient as indicated, passive exercises
- Maintains a healthy environment, including ensuring cleanliness of patient's immediate environment, laundering of patient's clothing, shopping to provide necessary food and sundries, planning and preparing meals, assisting patient in diversional activities, and providing simple treatments
- Reports significant data regarding the patient's condition or factors influencing the patient's welfare to the registered professional nurse
- Provides services as set forth in the plan of care

2. Homemaker services are provided by qualified homemakers in accordance with a plan of care prescribed by a physician, the written visit schedule, and written instructions from the supervising nurse or therapist. The homemaker carries out the following functions:
   - Provides minimal assistance with the patient's personal hygiene needs, including a partial bath, hair care, shaving, and dressing
   - Maintains a healthy environment, including ensuring cleanliness of patient's residence, laundering patient's clothes, shopping, preparing and serving meals, and performing other household chores
   - Reports significant data regarding the patient's condition or factors influencing the patient's welfare to the registered professional nurse
   - Provides services as set forth in the plan of care

3. The home health aide/homemaker completes the home health aide activity record on every visit and submits it to the supervisor.

4. The home health aide/homemaker reports immediately via phone any significant data regarding the patient's condition to a hospice team member, the home care department supervisor, the supervising nurse, or the therapist.

2. These measures constitute the scope of homemaker practice in a home care setting and comply with Medicare Conditions of Participation.

3. Documentation of care provided is mandated.

4. Patient safety must be ensured.

Origin Date: _____
Revised Date: _____
Approved Date: _____
Originator: _____
Distribution: _____

1:28
HOME HEALTH AIDE TRAINING, CERTIFICATION, AND COMPETENCY EVALUATION PROGRAM

PURPOSE:

To establish guidelines for the implementation of the home health aide training, certification, and competency evaluation program

RESPONSIBLE PERSONNEL:

Director of professional services, supervisor for staff development/quality assessment and improvement, home health aide supervisor

OBJECTIVES:

- To develop the home health aide training and competency evaluation program consistent with the Conditions of Participation (Section 1:27) as mandated by OBRA 1987 and the Foundation for Hospice and Homecare standard
- To implement a training and competency evaluation program with the intent of certifying home health aides under our employ
- To conduct the 75-hour training program, including 16 hours of supervised practical training
- To perform competency evaluation testing and verify competency of the home health aide prior to the aide performing a specific function
- To conduct yearly performance appraisals that reflect evaluation of competency skills.
- To conduct 12 hours of inservice training per calendar year for all certified home health aides

POLICY:

- AMHHC will conduct a training and competency evaluation program with the intent to certify employees as home health aides. The title "home health aide," as defined in Section 418.94, will only be used for those employees who have successfully completed the training program and competency evaluation testing. An individual who is found to be unsatisfactory in more than one of the required topics is not considered to have successfully passed competency evaluations as determined by a qualified individual.
- A qualified individual is an RN who possesses a minimum of two years of nursing experience, one year of which must be in the provision of home health care.
- The training program must be a minimum of 75 hours, including 16 hours of supervised practical training. Practical training must be with an individual but not necessarily with a patient. Sixteen hours of classroom training must precede the supervised practical training.
- Performance appraisals and competency evaluations will be completed annually.

- The agency will maintain documentation to verify that the training and competency evaluation program meets the requirements of the Conditions of Participation. The program will be based on the "Model Curriculum and Teaching Guide for the Instruction of the Homemaker-Home Health Aide," developed by the National Home Caring Council. The program will include the following subject areas:
  - communication skills
  - observation, reporting, and documentation of patient status and the care or services furnished
  - reading and recording temperature, pulse and respiration
  - basic infection control procedures
  - basic elements of body function and changes in body function that must be reported to the supervisor
  - maintenance of a clean, safe, and healthy environment
  - recognizing emergencies and understanding of emergency procedures
  - the physical, emotional, and developmental characteristics of the populations served by the home health agency, including the need for respect for the patient, his or her privacy, and his or her property
  - appropriate and safe techniques in personal hygiene and grooming, including bed, sponge, tub, or shower bath; shampoo in sink, tub, or bed; nail and skin care; and oral hygiene
  - safe transfer techniques and ambulation
  - normal range of motion and positioning
  - adequate nutrition and fluid intake
  - any other task that the home health agency may choose to have the home health aide perform
  - preventive health concepts, which will be integrated throughout the entire curriculum

PROCEDURE:

Action	Rationale
1. All applicants hired will attend a departmental and condensed hospital orientation. All contract home health aides will be oriented to the agency by the agency supervisor or clinical supervisor.	1. To provide an overview of the philosophy and day-to-day operation of the agency and to acquaint applicants with the required basic tasks.
2. All individuals hired will spend a minimum of one day of observation with an experienced employee.	2. To provide a realistic view of the tasks performed in the home setting.
3. All noncertified employees will complete a training course that includes 60 hours of classroom and 16 hours of supervised practical training. This course will follow the "Model Curriculum and Teaching Guide for the Instruction of the HM/HHA," developed by the National Home Caring Council. Attach-	3. To comply with the requirements for training for home caring accreditation.

ment A lists topics that will be included in the curriculum.

4. At the completion of the course, all aides will be tested to verify competence in the performance of a task prior to performing that task in a home setting. The agency will use the checklists for skills demonstration as prepared by the National Home Caring Council. That testing will include a 50-question written test, prepared by the agency. Passing grade will be 70.

5. All aides will receive a written performance appraisal annually. Skill competency will be verified on an annual basis. Home health aides servicing Medicare-certified home health agency patients will be supervised every two weeks by the primary nurse.

6. All homemaker-home health aides will receive a minimum of 12 hours of inservice training per calendar year. The inservice training may be furnished while the aide is giving care to patients. The 12-hour requirement will be prorated in the first year of employment.

7. Home health aides are in the probationary period during the training program. Failure to successfully complete the training will result in termination.

8. All test results from the training programs will become part of the personnel file. Upon successful completion of a course, aides will receive a home health aide certificate, a copy of which will also be part of the personnel file.

9. Home health aides will be encouraged to sit for the national certification examination.

10. The hospice is responsible for training and supervising the contracted home health aide on additional skills beyond the basic skills listed in the personnel file and in the home health agency's clinical record.

11. Training may be waived for individuals with experience equivalent to required training. A minimum of one year of experience in a position as a nursing

4. To comply with the home health agency training and competency evaluation program consistent with the Conditions of Participation (COP 484.36) as mandated by OBRA 1987.

5. To comply with hospital policy.

6. To comply with home health agency training and competency evaluation program.

7. To ensure that home health aides are certified to provide care to the Medicare patient.

8. To provide evidence that the employee has completed the required training program.

9. To provide the home health aide with national certification.

10. To comply with the Medicare Conditions of Participation.

11. To comply with the HHA training and competency evaluation program consistent with the Conditions of Participation, the National Home Caring Coun-

assistant or home health aide is required. A new employee hired with a home health aide certificate or a state nursing assistant certification will be competency tested. Competency testing will include a written test as well as a skills demonstration checklist, in the lab and field. Those areas found deficient will be reviewed prior to retesting of field competency.
12. An employee returning from a leave of absence (LOA) greater than six months must complete a skills laboratory review prior to providing in-home care.

cil, and the Joint Commission on Accreditation of Healthcare Organizations.

After certification and initial field competency evaluation, all aides will be evaluated yearly, in the field, using the agency's form for documentation. In addition, aides will be supervised in the field every two weeks on all Medicare cases and quarterly on all other cases.

ATTACHMENT A

Section I—Orientation to Homemaker-Home Health Aide Services, 4½ Hours

Unit A: Why Homemaker-Home Health Aide Services, 2½ Hours
- Course and Class Introductions
- The Need for Home Care
- Clients' Rights
- History and Background of Homemaker-Home Health Aide Services
- Overview of the Training

Unit B: The Role of the Homemaker-Home Health Aide, 1 Hour
- The Care Team
- Homemaker-Home Health Aide Tasks and Responsibilities
- The Homemaker-Home Health Aide on the Care Team

Unit C: How Agencies Make Services Available to Clients and Families, 1 Hour
- Organization of the Agency
- The Delivery of Service by the Agency
- The Plan of Care
- Responsibility of the Agency to the Homemaker-Home Health Aide

Section II—Understanding and Working with Various Client Populations, 19 Hours

Unit A: Communication, 2 Hours
- Concepts of Communication
- How the Homemaker-Home Health Aide Uses Communication

- How To Communicate Better
- Recording and Reporting Observations

Unit B: Understanding Basic Human Needs, 2½ Hours
- The Family
- Individual and Family Differences
- The Need for Homemaker-Home Health Aide Services

Unit C: Understanding and Working with Children, 3 Hours
- Growth and Development
- The Need for Homemaker-Home Health Aide Services
- Reactions of Children and Family Members to Stress
- Role of the Homemaker-Home Health Aide in Working with Children and Families under Stress
- Child Abuse and Neglect

Unit D: Understanding and Working with Older Clients, 4 Hours
- Facts, Figures, Myths, and Needs in Aging
- The Aging Process
- Special Considerations in Caring for the Elderly
- Emotional Health
- Elder Abuse and Neglect

Unit E: Understanding and Working with Clients Who Are Ill, 2 Hours
- Services for Clients Who Are Ill and Their Families
- Common Reactions to Illness
- Goals for the Care of Clients Who Are Ill
- Health Care Tasks

Unit F: Understand and Working with Clients with Disabilities, 2½ Hours
- Introduction
- Special Needs
- Alzheimer's Disease

Unit G: Mental Health and Mental Illness, 2 Hours
- Characteristics of Mental Health
- The Definition and Nature of Mental Illness
- Care of Clients with Mental Illness
- Role of Homemaker-Home Health Aide in Situation Where There is Mental Illness
- Suicide

Unit H: Understanding Dying and Death, 1 Hour
- Behavior and Feelings about Death
- Caring for the Dying

Section III—Practical Knowledge and Skills in Home Management, 14½ Hours

Unit A: Maintaining a Clean, Safe, and Healthy Environment, 4½ Hours

- Contribution of Housekeeping and Maintenance to Physical and Psychological Well-Being
- Responsibilities of the Homemaker-Home Health Aide for Maintaining a Clean, Safe and Healthy Environment
- General Guidelines for Cleaning a House
- Cleaning and Maintaining Clothing
- Teaching Others To Assist in or Do Home Maintenance

Unit B: Food and Nutrition, 6 Hours
- Importance of Food and Nutrition
- Meal Planning
- Food Shopping
- Meal Preparation
- Proper Food Storage, Food Sanitation, and Kitchen Safety
- Nutritional Problems of the Aged and Ill
- Modified Diets

Unit C: Managing Time, Energy, Money, and Other Resources, 2 Hours
- Time and Energy Management
- Use of Resources
- Money Management

Unit D: Home Maintenance When Disease is Present, 2 Hours
- Infectious Diseases
- Infection Control
- Acquired Immune Deficiency Syndrome (AIDS)

Section IV—Practical Knowledge and Skills in Personal Care, 22 hours

Unit A: Body Systems, Disorders, and Disease, 3 Hours
- Overview of the Body
- Body Systems

Unit B: Observing Body Functions, 3 Hours
- Signs and Symptoms of Illness
- Temperature, Pulse, and Respiration
- Urine Test for Sugar

Unit C: Care of the Client in Bed, 8-1/2 hours
- Introduction
- Body Mechanics
- Positioning the Client Who Is Ill
- Elimination of Body Waste
- Bathing and Grooming
- Changing Bed Linens

Unit D: Care of the Client Not Confined to Bed, 1½ hours
- Getting the Client out of Bed
- Getting the Client up in a Chair

- Helping a Client To Walk
- Hygiene and Grooming for the Ambulatory Client

Unit E: Observations about Medications, 1 hour
- General Information about Medications
- Role of the Homemaker-Home Health Aide
- Observations, Reporting, and Safety
- Storage of Medications
- Drug Misuse
- Safe Use of Oxygen

Unit F: Rehabilitation, 2 hours
- Needs of the Client with Limited Function
- Range of Motion Exercises
- The Client with One-Sided Weakness
- Assistive Devices
- Adapting the Environment

Unit G: Health and Emergency Procedures, 3 hours
- Dry, Nonsterile Technique Dressings
- Simple Procedures
- General Guidelines for Handling Emergencies
- Responding in an Emergency

Basic Vocabulary
- Preventive health concepts are integrated throughout the entire curriculum.

Origin Date: _____
Revised Date: _____
Approved Date: _____
Originator: _____
Distribution: _____

1:29
HOSPICE/HOME CARE VOLUNTEERS

PURPOSE:

To establish guidelines for volunteer services

RESPONSIBLE PERSONNEL:

Executive director, director of professional services, director of hospice/home care volunteers

OBJECTIVES:

- To establish guidelines for hospice/home care volunteer services for hospital patients not currently enrolled in AMH home care services

- To initiate volunteer services to terminally ill patients who are still in the hospital but will become hospice/home care patients when discharged
- To provide continued volunteer service to hospice/home care patients who are admitted to the hospital
- To use volunteers effectively and efficiently within their scope of responsibility

POLICY:

Hospice/home care volunteers function under the general guidance of the director of volunteers of the hospice/home care program with regard to time, assignment, conduct, and policy. Volunteers may be assigned to hospital patients who will benefit from the relationship prior to hospital discharge. Volunteers assigned to hospice/home care patients provide continuity by continuing to visit patients admitted to the hospital. When a hospice/home care volunteer is assigned to visit a patient on a hospital nursing unit, the volunteer is responsible to the nurse manager or his or her designee for procedures and quality of performance. The volunteer functions as a support to the patient and as a friendly visitor.

PROCEDURE:

Action	Rationale
1. Hospital staff identify patients who would benefit from volunteer service while still in the hospital and notify a hospital case manager.	1. Hospital staff are most aware of patient needs.
2. The case manager notifies the director of hospice/home care volunteers, who assigns a volunteer.	2. The director knows the skills of the volunteers and can match them to the needs of the patient.

Hospice Patient Admitted to Hospital

Action	Rationale
1. Hospice coordinator notifies appropriate team members of patient admission to hospital.	1. Communication ensures coordination of care among hospice team members and inpatient staff.
2. The hospice case manager develops a hospice plan of care to determine inpatient services.	2. The program meets Medicare Conditions of Participation.
3. The director of volunteers notifies the volunteer of the proposed visit schedule and revised plan of care.	3. The director of volunteers is responsible for assigning volunteers and monitoring their performance.
4. The volunteer wears identification badge and signs in at the hospital volunteer office.	4. Personnel working with patients should always be identifiable.
5. The volunteer will report to the patient's primary nurse when arriving on the unit and when leaving the unit.	5. The volunteer identifies him- or herself to hospital staff.
6. The volunteer communicates any pertinent information gained while relating to the patient to hospice team members.	6. Communication ensures coordination.

7. The volunteer completes required documentation related to service provided and time.	7. The volunteer is an important member of the care team. Information needs to be communicated to other team members. Volunteer time is credited to the volunteer and the program.

Origin Date: _____
Revised Date: _____
Approved Date: _____
Originator: _____
Distribution: _____

1:30
HOPICE PATIENTS RESIDING IN PERSONAL CARE OR SKILLED NURSING FACILITIES

PURPOSE:

To establish policy and procedures for the provision of hospice benefit services to patients in personal care facilities (PCFs), or skilled nursing facilities (SNFs), with consideration for all staff

RESPONSIBLE PERSONNEL:

All members of hospice interdisciplinary team, PCF staff, SNF staff

POLICY:

Abington Memorial Hospital's Home Care Hospice Program is available to provide Medicare hospice benefit services to eligible residents of PCFs and SNFs. A resident is considered eligible if he or she has available Medicare Part A (Medicare is not providing for room and board), the patient has an illness certified by a physician as terminal (a life expectancy of six months or less), and the patient/family and physician request palliative care.

PROCEDURE:

Action	Rationale
1. Patients will be admitted to the PCF/SNF prior to hospice start of care.	1. This provides for a smooth Medicare billing cycle.
2. Hospice will provide durable medical equipment (DME) with physician's order and arrange delivery/pickup.	2. DME is provided through hospice benefit by hospice contract company.
• Any other DME requirements will need to be called to hospice by PCF/SNF staff.	• Medicare billing is not available should the PCF/SNF provide the patient with DME.
3. PCF/SNF staff, position, and hospice team members need to coordinate any laboratory or other diagnostic tests.	3. Coordination ensures that procedures are palliative in nature. The patient and/or PCF/SNF is financially responsible for

4. PCF/SNF staff, position, and hospice team coordinate symptom management.
   a. Hospice nurse is called by PCF/SNF staff with any problems.
   b. A plan is suggested and physician is phoned by hospice nurse.
   c. Physician phones PCF/SNF nurse with necessary verbal orders.
   d. If patient's primary physician is unavailable, hospice medical director is phoned.

5. A flyer is posted on patient's medical record, which includes the hospice name, primary nurse's name, and the emergency service members.

6. Hospice nurse will document significant findings in PCF/SNF clinical record.

lab tests/procedures not approved by hospice team.

4. All staff members' input is necessary to ensure quality hospice care.
   a. Hospice emergency service is available 24 hours a day.
   b. Terminal symptom management is the hospice nurses' area of expertise.
   c. To meet PCF/SNF regulatory guidelines.
   d. Medical director is also an authorized physician able to participate in plan of care and order necessary changes.

5. To ensure coordination and communication among staff and shifts.

6. To promote communication among disciplines and staff.

Origin Date: _____
Revised Date: _____
Approved Date: _____
Originator: _____
Distribution: _____

1:31
HOSPICE SUPPORT GROUP

- A support group is available for the hospice team members to address issues such as staff stress, grieving, and clinical needs. The group is open to all professional team members and meets at the discretion of the hospice coordinator, or at least quarterly. The hospice IDG may initiate a request for additional support services. If need arises, administration will consider the support group's request for additional external stress management and/or bereavement resources.
- Emphasis will be placed on the use of the support group as a constructive means to reduce stress associated with hospice patient care and to promote research in the area of stress management and patient care.
- In addition to the hospice support group, the AMH employee assistance program is available to provide individual counseling as indicated.

Origin Date: _____
Revised Date: _____
Approved Date: _____
Originator: _____
Distribution: _____

1:32
INCIDENT REPORTING

PURPOSE:

To provide systematic documentation of all unusual incidents

RESPONSIBLE PERSONNEL:

Executive director, all staff

OBJECTIVES:

- To establish a systematic/standardized documentation process for all unusual incidents
- To provide a record of occurrences as a basis for notification to the insurance carrier in anticipation of potential litigation
- To provide a database for the organization to evaluate type and cause of incidents, to institute corrective measures to improve risk management and quality of care, and to reduce recurring incidents
- To provide a mechanism for evaluation of the safety and infection control program and the tracking and trending of safety and infection control problems
- To provide a mechanism for tracking of sentinel events

POLICY:

- An incident report is completed by any employee who performs, discovers, witnesses, or becomes aware of circumstances indicative of an event. An incident is defined as any happening that is not consistent with the routine operation of the organization or the routine care of the patient and that has a potential litigious aspect or may compromise patient care, such as the following:
  - loss or breakage
  - endangerment of staff or patients
  - untoward outcomes, including drug reactions, IV therapy complications, infections
  - motor vehicle accident
  - staff infections
  - equipment or medical device failure
  - procedure error that results in trauma or injury
  - patient/staff falls
  - medication error*
  - staff accidents resulting in injury
  - patient/family complaint
- The purpose of the incident report is to provide a prompt and accurate account of an event, a method for discovery and investigation of causes, to facilitate notification of the insurance carrier, and to provide data for evaluation and prevention of incidents. All reports are to be completed in an objective, factual, and nonaccusatory manner. Incident reports are not used for punitive measures or as a basis for disciplinary actions.

PROCEDURE:

Action	Rationale
1. The person performing, witnessing, or becoming aware of circumstances indicative of an event documents the inci-	1. All employees are responsible for reporting promptly and accurately all events they become aware of, whether or not

---

*Medication errors are defined as medication administered by nurse without order, incorrect dosage, improper order, incorrect drug, duplication, incorrect mode of administration, omission, patient took unprescribed medication, or dispensing error by pharmacy.

dent in writing on the standardized incident reporting form as promptly and accurately as possible following the occurrence. The incident report form defines the types of accidents, injuries, and safety hazards to be reported.
2. All medically relevant events happening to patients shall be documented in the patient's record, but the fact that an incident report has been filed shall not be documented in the patient's record.
3. The incident report is forwarded to the employee's supervisor and then to the director of professional services for signature and on to the director of risk management within 72 hours of occurrence of the event. The supervisor is responsible for instituting corrective action when indicated.
4. The supervisor or director of professional services notifies the director of risk management immediately by phone of any urgent or critical incident.
5. The director of professional services gives priority to all reports involving serious injury and/or potential litigation, that is, sentinel events. The director sets in motion appropriate action to investigate the event. This may include, but is not limited to, discussion with the personnel involved, the person's supervisor, the attending physician, and, if indicated, the patient. All discussion is documented. Prompt notification is made to the insurance carrier.
6. All other incident reports are reviewed, analyzed, and trended by the director of professional services.
7. Incident reports that indicate that an infection developed as a result of care will be analyzed and handled according to policy. The incidence of an infection will have been reported to the physician.
8. Individual supervisors and the director of professional services monitor incident reports and summaries of trends on a periodic basis. As the hospital incident report contains limited information for

they were directly involved. Reporting is done in writing to provide data for the insurance carrier and for organizational analysis and prevention.

2. Documentation of medically relevant events in the patient record is sufficient legally. This is to protect against undue litigation for the organization.

3. Timely submission of reports promotes timely investigation of the incident and any indicated action.

4. Timely submission of reports promotes timely investigation of the incident and any indicated action.

5. Prompt investigation and reporting of sentinel events provides data in case of future claim activity or litigious action. Examples of sentinel events are anaphylaxis secondary to medication administration, injuries attributable to direct patient care, and staff injuries resulting in hospitalization.

6. This analysis identifies system problems, educational needs, or needed procedural changes.

7. This analysis is needed to meet Joint Commission and regulatory requirements.

8. Monitoring of trends on a periodic basis provides an indication of the quality of care relative to that service and forms a basis for any needed action, including inservice programs.

tracking, staff will also be instructed to complete the Departmental Incident Tracking Form (Form 9).

9. The director of risk management forwards summary reports periodically to the executive director.

9. The reports are evaluated for trends and identification of needed organization-wide corrective measures.

Origin Date: _____
Revised Date: _____
Approved Date: _____
Originator: _____
Distribution: _____

1:33
INFECTION CONTROL: UNIVERSAL BLOOD AND BODY FLUID PRECAUTIONS

PURPOSE:

To prevent the transmission of bloodborne pathogens

RESPONSIBLE PERSONNEL:

Executive director, director of professional services, supervisors, and clinical staff. Department heads and supervisory personnel are responsible for reviewing this policy with employees who are classified as having potential exposure to blood or other potentially infective material. Director of education and staff development or designee in consultation with AMH infection control practitioners is responsible for inservice education programs.

OBJECTIVES:

- To develop and implement infection control procedures
- To establish infection control standards in compliance with Centers for Disease Control (CDC) and the Occupational Safety and Health Act (OSHA) requirements

POLICY:

Medical history and examination cannot reliably identify all patients infected with Human Immunodeficiency Virus (HIV) or other bloodborne pathogens, therefore blood and fluid precautions should be consistently used for *all* patients. This approach, which has been recommended by the CDC and is referred to as "universal blood and body fluid precautions," should be used in the care of *all* patients. Infection control standards are established in compliance with the recommendations of the CDC in Atlanta and OSHA. Staff who are at risk for exposure are educated to these standards and they are practiced consistently. Any incidents of infection related to care and services are reported according to Policy 1:34.

PROCEDURE:

Action	Rationale
1. Staff are oriented to general infection control procedures upon employment. On-going training is conducted annually thereafter.	1. Compliance with OSHA Part 1910 Section 1910.1030 of Title 29 of the Code of Federal Regulations.
2. The home care staff are oriented to the universal blood and body precautions as established by OSHA and the CDC. These work practices are carried out during patient care as follows:	
A. Handwashing requirements	
1. Handwashing is required before and after contact with all patients using an antiseptic microbial skin cleanser.	Compliance with OSHA Part 1910 Section 1910.1030 of Title 29 of the Code of Federal Regulations.
2. Handwashing facilities are generally available in most patients homes. In the event that facilities are not available staff will cleanse their hands with an alcohol-based handwashing solution. Hands must be thoroughly washed with soap and water as soon as facilities are available.	Prevents transmission by direct or indirect contact with the source of an infection such as purulent drainage, etc. Protects patients and clients with compromised immunity.
B. Gloves	
1. Gloves must be worn for any contact with blood or body fluids, mucous membranes, or non-intact skin of all patients and for handling items or surfaces soiled with blood or body fluids.	
2. Gloves should always be worn for vascular access procedures, including phlebotomy.	
3. Gloves should be replaced as soon as possible if they are torn, punctured, or when their integrity is compromised.	
4. Single-use gloves shall not be washed or decontaminated for re-use.	
5. Staff shall wash hands and any other potentially contaminated skin area with soap and water immediately or as soon as feasible after removing gloves.	

6. Employees who have allergic reactions to gloves should be evaluated in AMH Employee/Student Health. Appropriate alternatives shall be made readily accessible.
7. Employees who have exudative lesions or weeping dermatitis should refrain from all direct patient care and from handling patient-care equipment until the condition resolves. These employees should be referred to AMH Employee/Student Health.
8. Gloves must be discarded after contact with each patient.

C. Personnel protective equipment
1. Masks and eye protection should be worn during procedures that are likely to generate splashes, sprays, or droplets of potentially infectious material that may come in contact with eyes, nose, or mouth. Masks should also be worn to protect against transmission of airborne infection such as TB and influenza.
2. Fluid resistant gowns or aprons should be worn during procedures that are likely to generate splashes of blood or body fluids or when there is the potential for soilage of caregivers clothing with patients blood, body fluid, or stool.
3. To minimize the need for emergency mouth-to-mouth resuscitation, resuscitation masks shall be available for use. The resuscitation masks are contained in the nursing bag and are given to the nurse during orientation. The masks are disposed after one use and shall be immediately replaced.
4. All personal protective equipment shall be removed, double bagged, secured, and discarded as household waste.
5. If personal protective equipment is penetrated by blood or other potentially infectious materials, it should

Compliance with OSHA Part 1910 Section 1910.1030 of Title 29 of the Code of Federal Regulations.

Prevents transmission by direct or indirect contact with the source of an infection such as purulent drainage, etc.

Protects patients and clients with compromised immunity.

be removed as soon as feasible and discarded.
6. All personal protective equipment will be provided, and replaced by AMHHC at no cost to employees. Nurses will carry their protective equipment in their bags which are taken into the patient's home.
7. Disposable personal protective equipment is obtained from the AMH storeroom and various home care vendors. Supply room clerk and department managers are responsible for ensuring that an adequate supply of personal protective equipment is available.

D. Post-contact cleansing requirements
1. Hands and other skin surfaces should be washed immediately and thoroughly with soap and water if contaminated with blood or other moist body substances.
2. Mucous membranes should be flushed with water immediately or as soon as feasible following contact with blood or other potentially infectious materials.
3. Hands should be washed immediately after gloves are removed.
4. Antiseptic towelettes or alcohol-based handwashing solutions may be used as temporary substitutes for handwashing. Hands should be washed with soap and water as soon as feasible.

E. Contaminated sharps
1. All employees should take precautions to prevent injuries caused by needles, scalpels, and other sharp items
    a. during procedures
    b. during disposal of used needles
    c. when handling sharp instruments after procedures.
2. To prevent needlestick injuries:
    a. used needles should not be recapped or removed from syringes.
    b. used needles may not be bent, broken, sheared, or manipulated

Prevents the transmission of infection.

Protects patients and clients with compromised immunity.

Compliance with OSHA Part 1910 Section 1910.1030 of Title 29 of the Code of Federal Regulations.

by hand.
   c. used lancets are to be removed from the lancet device with a hemostat.
   d. after use, disposable syringes and needles, scalpel blades, and other sharp items must be placed in appropriate containers for disposal. These containers must be:
      - puncture resistant
      - red in color and labeled "Biohazard"
      - leakproof on the sides and bottom
      - able to be securely closed
      - closed prior to removal or replacement to prevent spillage or protrusion of contents during handling or transport
      - maintained in an upright position while in use
      - replaced routinely and not allowed to over fill
   e. Puncture-resistant containers will be left in the patient's home for use by the nurse.
   f. Filled containers will be double bagged in a red biohazard bag and transported back to the agency for disposal.
   g. The double bagged container will be placed in a large red biohazard container for disposal by outside vendor.
3. Patient education regarding disposal of sharps.
   a. Patients are instructed on proper disposal of sharps as per the recommendations of the United States Environmental Protection Agency (USEPA) and Pennsylvania Department of Environmental Resources (PA-DER).
   b. Refer to USEPA Document *Disposal Tips for Home Health Care*.

F. Lab Specimens
   1. Blood and urine specimens are generally collected and transported by AMA laboratory technicians.

2. In the event that the hospice nurse is required to collect and transport specimens, the specimen will be placed in a container marked "Biohazard" for transport to the hospital.
3. If the outside surface of a specimen container is soiled or likely to be soiled, the container should be secured in a plastic bag. Plastic bags should be available in the nurse's or laboratory technician's bag.

G. Equipment
1. Disposable supplies and equipment are recommended for home use. Prior to issuance of supplies, staff checks for expiration dates. Clean and sterile supplies are maintained in manufacturer's packaging for transport to the patient's home.
2. Vacutainers will be provided for the patient and then discarded.
3. Reusable equipment if soiled with infectious material shall be cleaned and sanitized with a phenolic solution or 1:10 bleach solution. *Note:* Baby scales are cleaned with a phenolic solution after each use. During use, scales are covered with a protective barrier.
4. If the potential for exposure to infectious material exists sphygmomanometers should be placed over a dry skin area which has been covered with a layer of material. The diaphragm of the stethoscope should be cleaned with alcohol wipes, then when feasible sanitized with a phenolic solution.
5. Phenolic solution in ready to use containers can be obtained from the environmental services department or supply room.

H. Housekeeping requirements
1. All equipment and environmental work surfaces that have had contact with blood or other potentially infectious materials shall be cleaned with a detergent and disinfected

Compliance with OSHA Part 1910 Section 1910.1030 of Title 29 of the Code of Federal Regulations.

with a phenolic solution or 1:10 bleach solution.
   a. Phenolic solution in ready to use containers can be obtained from the environmental services department or supply room.
2. Broken glass which may be contaminated shall not be picked up directly with hands. It must be cleaned up using mechanical means such as a brush and dust pan, tongs, or forceps.
3. Management of spills of blood or other potentially infectious materials.
   a. Spills may be cleaned using appropriate personal protective equipment. The spill should be cleaned with a household detergent then disinfected with a phenolic or 1:10 bleach solution.
   b. Protective coverings such as plastic wrap, foil, or imperviously backed absorbent paper used to cover equipment and environmental services shall be removed and replaced as soon as feasible when they become contaminated.

I. Laundry
   1. Soiled linens contaminated with infectious material shall be handled as little as possible with a minimum of agitation.
   2. Soiled linens shall be bagged at the location where it was used and transported to the laundry room.

J. Communication of hazards to employees
   1. Labels and signs
      a. Utilizing universal precautions for the handling of all specimens, the labeling/color coding of specimens is not necessary provided containers are recognizable as containing specimens.
      b. Warning labels employing the fluorescent orange symbol for biohazard shall be affixed to containers used to store or trans-

Compliance with OSHA Part 1910 Section 1910.1030 of Title 29 of the Code of Federal Regulations.

port potentially infectious materials.
   c. Red bags or red containers may be used to designate infectious waste as specified in the AMH waste management policy.
K. General requirements
   1. Eating, drinking, smoking, applying cosmetics or lip balm, and handling contact lenses are prohibited in homes where there is reasonable likelihood of exposure to blood or body fluids.
L. Pregnant health-care workers are not known to be at greater risk of contracting HIV, HBV, or other bloodborne infections than health-care workers who are not pregnant. However, if a health-care worker develops a blood-borne infection during pregnancy, the infant is at risk of infection resulting from perinatal transmission. Because of this risk, pregnant employees should be especially familiar with and strictly adhere to universal blood and body fluid precautions.

Compliance with OSHA Part 1910 Section 1910.1030 of Title 29 of the Code of Federal Regulations.

Origin Date: _____
Revised Date: _____
Approved Date: _____
Originator: _____
Distribution: _____

1:34
INFECTION CONTROL TRACKING AND REPORTING

PURPOSE:

To establish protocols for the tracking, reporting, and analyzing of infections

RESPONSIBLE PERSONNEL:

Director of professional services, supervisors, clinical staff

OBJECTIVE:

To delineate agency procedure for tracking, reporting, and analyzing infections

POLICY:

- As per the requirements of the Joint Commission, Abington Memorial Hospital Home Care (AMHHC) will report, evaluate, and maintain records of infections related to care/

service. This will be accomplished by a twofold process. As part of the quality assessment and improvement program, studies will be conducted of infections in select populations of patients. In addition to the formal study, staff are instructed to track select infections, substantiated by positive cultures, which occurred during the home care course of treatment.
- Any staff infection resulting from a work-related incident must immediately be reported to the employee health department.

PROCEDURE:

Action	Rationale
1. The director of quality assessment and improvement will conduct a study of infection rates in select populations.	1. Population to study may be determined by general tracking.
2. Staff are requested to report on an incident report any infections substantiated by positive cultures and a temperature greater than 100°, and in which antibiotics are prescribed, which occurred during the home care course of treatment.	2. Direction will be provided to staff to assist them in focusing tracking. Select areas may be targeted in any given year.
3. Incident reports are reviewed and kept on file.	3. Recordkeeping provides a mechanism to track infections.
4. An analysis of the infection reports will be conducted annually.	4. This analysis forms the basis for determination of areas that need further study by the director of quality assessment and improvement.
5. Staff are informed of the outcomes.	5. The goal is to improve patient care.
6. Staff infections: staff are required to complete an employee accident and illness report (in lieu of an incident report). The report is forwarded to the AMHHC administrative staff for review and analysis, then forwarded to employee health.	6. The employee health department is responsible for protecting the health of employees.

Origin Date: _____
Revised Date: _____
Approved Date: _____
Originator: _____
Distribution: _____

1:35
INTAKE PROCEDURE

PURPOSE:

To establish procedure for acceptance of referrals

RESPONSIBLE PERSONNEL:

Receptionist, supervisory staff, clinical staff, discharge planning nurses, intake nurses

OBJECTIVES:

- To designate the organization's protocol for acceptance of referrals
- To delineate responsibilities for personnel involved in intake

POLICY:

Personnel are available to accept referrals 24 hours per day.

PROCEDURE:

Action	Rationale
1. The organization has incoming telephone lines that ring in sequence.	1. Numbers to access hospice care services are publicized to the community. There are multiple lines to prevent long waits for referring sources.
2. During scheduled working hours, calls are transferred to the intake nurse and/or clinical supervisor, who obtains initial patient care information.	2. The referral source communicates patient information directly to a professional nurse. Physician orders can be obtained immediately if referral is from a physician.
3. The intake nurse, in collaboration with the supervisor, determines if the department can provide service. If service can be provided, the intake nurse or supervisor accepts referral information and completes the intake form. If the call is not from a physician, the physician is contacted to confirm service needs and to obtain a verbal order. If service cannot be provided, the caller is given names of other agencies that can provide required services.	3. A physician's order is required prior to start of care.
4. The supervisor assigns cases to individual professional or support staff based on patient need and level of care required, geographical area, and qualifications of staff needed.	4. Supervisor considers numerous factors in assigning cases to appropriate staff. This enables the department to provide the highest quality of services consistent with patient needs.
5. The nurse is responsible for coordination of services the patient receives from referral to discharge.	5. Department practices a system of primary nursing and makes every effort to keep the attending physician apprised of patient status.
6. After scheduled hours (weekends and evenings), one published number is attached to an automatic answering ma-	6. Enables referral source to have 24-hour access to services.

chine. A caller can leave a message that will be taken off the tape the next morning.

7. The taped message informs the caller to dial the listed number, which is answered by a 24-hour answering service if immediate service is needed.
8. A fax machine is available to the discharge planning nurses in the hospital for transmitting referral information directly to the office.
9. Fax referrals must be preceded by a telephone call to the supervisor or nurse on call.

7. The registered nurse is available to answer questions, offer telephone reassurance, or make necessary home visits.

8. The fax machine allows for communication of detailed information directly to the caregiver, which decreases the amount of time spent on phone referrals.

9. A telephone call preceding the fax informs staff of a pending referral and possible need for home visit when the office is not open.

Origin Date: _____
Revised Date: _____
Approved Date: _____
Originator: _____
Distribution: _____

**1:36
INTERDISCIPLINARY GROUP**

POLICY:
- The hospice program consists of the following members on a regular basis:
  - hospice coordinator/clinical nursing supervisor
  - medical director
  - medical social worker
  - director of volunteers
  - chaplain—pastoral counselor
  - hospice primary nurse
  - inpatient hospice case manager
- The following members are added for individual patients, as appropriate:
  - physical therapist
  - occupational therapist
  - speech pathologist
  - volunteers
  - home health aides
  - psychiatric nurse
  - registered dietician
- The IDG shall meet at least biweekly whenever there are active hospice patients on the AMHHC Hospice Program to evaluate patient status, participate in problem solving, and plan for patients' care needs.
- The hospice program has designated a registered nurse to coordinate the implementation of the plan of care for each patient.

- The hospice coordinator/clinical nursing supervisor acts as a consultant to the hospice nursing staff regarding clinical management of the hospice patient. The coordinator/supervisor or designee presides at team meetings and is responsible for recording the IDG plan of care updates and team conference notes.

Origin Date: _____
Revised Date: _____
Approved Date: _____
Originator: _____
Distribution: _____

1:37
INTERDISCIPLINARY GROUP COORDINATION

OBJECTIVES:

To exercise a coordinated effort for the provision of comprehensive hospice care to meet the health needs of the hospice patients and families

METHODOLOGY:

Provide for mutual participation with interdisciplinary group (IDG), family/patient, and all appropriate available health disciplines to:
1. Confine all available services to this hospice rather than share with others providing like services.
2. Assess, explore, and plan for the required services.
3. Determine levels and types of required services, including continuous care, acute care, respite, and home care.
4. Establish realistic goals.
5. Coordinate with all involved services to unify and maximize their contributions.
6. Establish a plan of care and visitation schedule.
7. Communicate in planned weekly IDG meetings and spontaneous conferences to evaluate progress and consider revision of goals to meet changing needs.
8. Document visits and IDG team conferences, provision of therapeutic care, achievement of progress, and other pertinent data.
9. Audit services for quality care, including the provision of therapeutic measures, need for added services or termination of same, revision of visit schedule, and so forth.
10. Revise for follow-up or referral upon termination of services or when need identified. Referral is made to the appropriate source, such as nutrition support, psychiatric clinician, or respite by the interdisciplinary group.

Origin Date: _____
Revised Date: _____
Approved Date: _____
Originator: _____
Distribution: _____

1:38
INTERDISCIPLINARY PLAN OF CARE

- The interdisciplinary team care plan is developed for each patient/family based on clinical information in the initial assessment by at least three members of the IDG.
- The care plan documents
  - identified patient/family problems and needs, including the management of discomfort and symptom relief
  - identified goals that are realistic, achievable, and measurable
  - care and services, including medications prescribed and medical equipment required to be provided to meet the identified goals
  - the signatures of the attending physician, team coordinator and medical director
- Verbal orders are signed by the attending physician when an additional discipline enters the patient/family care or when there is a change in management.
- The interdisciplinary plan of care is reviewed on a regular basis by the IDG during weekly team conferences. Each patient is reviewed and his or her plan of care updated at least every two weeks. Documentation of the review and update will be recorded in the team conference notes, signed by team coordinator and medical director, with changes forwarded to attending physician via verbal orders.

Origin Date: _____
Revised Date: _____
Approved Date: _____
Originator: _____
Distribution: _____

1:39
LETTER OF EXPLANATION FOR FUNERAL DIRECTORS

Dear Funeral Director:

The patient named below is terminally ill and has chosen, with the help of the family and physician, to remain at home until death. The family has chosen your funeral home and will be contacting you to arrange services. Abington Memorial Hospital Home Care Hospice Program is providing hospice care and support to the patient and family in the terminal stage of illness. This letter is to acquaint you with hospice procedures at the time of death so that we may better work with you to support and help the family.

Our goal is to prepare the family, teaching them what to expect and what needs to be done at the time of death. We encourage families to make funeral arrangements in advance and to have a list of telephone numbers available. The hospice on-call nurse helps the family notify the physician and funeral director and provides other support as needed.

As you no doubt know, Pennsylvania has no law stating that a body must be pronounced dead. The patient's physician, named below, has agreed to sign the death certificate and must be contacted by the funeral director to arrange completion of the certification within the required 96 hours.

If you have any questions or if we can be of any help to you, please call me at the below number any weekday between 8:30 A.M. and 5:00 P.M. Thank you for your help in providing support to our patient and family.

Sincerely,

Hospice Clinical Supervisor

Patient's Name: _____ Phone: _____
Address: _____

Responsible Family Member: _____ Phone: _____
Address: _____

Primary Physician: _____ Phone: _____
Address: _____

Origin Date: _____
Revised Date: _____
Approved Date: _____
Originator: _____
Distribution: _____

1:40
LEVELS OF CARE

OBJECTIVE:

To delegate qualified personnel to provide services in accordance with prescribed treatment and individual patient needs

POLICY:

I. Routine Home Care

Hospice services, including all interdisciplinary group members and drugs and biologicals for hospice benefit patients are available for routine home care. The focus of care is management of patient symptoms and support and counseling to patients and families in the home. This level of care requires intermittent home visits. The primary caregiver is responsible for the patient's care during the intervals between hospice home visits. Intensity and frequency of visits are based on the individual's needs.

II. Continuous Care

During periods of crisis, nursing care is available for as much as 24 hours a day or as necessary to maintain an individual at home. Either homemaker or home health aide, or both, may be provided during periods of crisis, but care during periods of crisis must be predominantly nursing care. A period of crisis is a period in which the individual requires continuous care to achieve palliation or management of acute medical symptoms. This level of care may be covered by Medicare hospice benefits or other third-party payers.

III. Inpatient Care (Acute)

Inpatient care for acute patient management is available at Abington Memorial Hospital for patients covered by the Medicare hospice benefit or at the hospital of the patient's (and physician's) choice for other third-party payers. The hospice provides the inpatient facility a copy of the patient plan of care and specifies the inpatient services to be furnished.

IV. Inpatient Care (Respite)

Inpatient care for respite of patient and primary care providers is available for hospice benefit patients per contracts. Respite care for other patients may be available through their third-party payers or through other resources available to the home care department.

Origin Date: _____
Revised Date: _____
Approved Date: _____
Originator: _____
Distribution: _____

1:41
LICENSURE AND CERTIFICATION VERIFICATION

PURPOSE:

To ensure that all professional and contract personnel have current licenses and certification verification, when applicable

RESPONSIBLE PERSONNEL:

Executive director, supervisors, administrative assistant

OBJECTIVE:

To maintain Medicare and Joint Commission accreditation in keeping all licenses and registrations up-to-date in all clinical areas

POLICY:

The organization requires verification of licensure and certification at least every year upon renewal.

PROCEDURE:

Action	Rationale
1. Verify that all professional employees and personnel under arrangement and contract have current licenses and/or required certification.	1. These documents are evidence that Joint Commission, Medicare, and agency standards are met.

2. Call or write the State Board of Nursing with license information.
3. Keep records and input data into computer system for all professional and contract personnel, noting due dates for renewal of licenses.
4. Notify personnel/contractors when new copies of licenses are due to keep agency files up-to-date.
5. Incorporate current documents into personnel or contract file.
6. File professional certification documents when presented.

2. All professional licenses are current.
3. Data printout verifies that all information is current.
4. Joint Commission, Medicare, and agency requirements are met.
5. Personnel files include pertinent documents.
6. Acknowledge all credentials that staff/contractors have acquired.

Origin Date: _____
Revised Date: _____
Approved Date: _____
Originator: _____
Distribution: _____

1:42
MEDICAL DEVICE REPORTING

PURPOSE:

To develop and implement medical device reporting procedures

RESPONSIBLE PERSONNEL:

Administration, supervisory staff, clinical and contract staff, durable medical equipment (DME) companies

OBJECTIVES:

- To provide identification, communication, and evaluation of events that may be subject to medical device reporting
- To establish a review procedure
- To ensure that medical device reports are submitted to manufacturer and the Food and Drug Administration (FDA), as per hospital policy

POLICY:

- The Safe Medical Device Act requires home health agencies to report device-related deaths or serious injury to the manufacturer of the device involved or the FDA within 10 days of their becoming aware of an incident.
- Since Abington Memorial Hospital Home Care (AMHHC) is not a direct supplier of durable medical equipment, the DME company that provided the equipment to the patient is responsible for meeting this requirement. In the event that a device-related death or serious injury occurs secondary to equipment directly provided by AMHHC, the department will follow the hospital's procedure. The biomedical engineering department will be contacted immediately to investigate the event and provide direction.

DEFINITION:

Serious injury is defined as a serious illness or injury that is life threatening, results in permanent damage to a body structure, or necessitates immediate medical or surgical intervention to preclude permanent impairment of a body function or permanent damage to a body structure.

PROCEDURE:

Action	Rationale
1. Staff and contractors are required to complete an incident report for malfunctioning of any equipment such as DME, infusion pumps, intravenous catheters, and any other catheters.	1. A medical device can cause or contribute to a reportable event in several ways, including failure, malfunction, faulty design, or labeling and user error.
2. The nurse, therapist, or supervisor reports malfunction of DME to the supplier of the equipment.	2. AMHHC is not a direct provider of DME. The DME companies provide equipment directly for the patient and bill a client's insurance.
3. In the event of serious injury or death related to equipment malfunction, the biomedical engineering department will be consulted and the DME company will be notified.	3. The biomedical engineering department will provide guidance and direction. An incident report will be completed.
4. In addition to the hospital, the home care department will maintain medical device reporting files.	4. The department will follow the incident report tracking policy.

Origin Date: _____
Revised Date: _____
Approved Date: _____
Originator: _____
Distribution: _____

1:43
MEDICAL SERVICES PLAN OF CARE

PURPOSE:

To establish criteria for the medical services to patients/families

RESPONSIBLE PERSONNEL:

Professional advisory committee, executive director, director of professional services

OBJECTIVES:

- To establish the requirements for the physician's plan of treatment for all patients
- To establish standards for physicians' supervision of care

POLICY:

- All patients serviced by the home care service must be under medical supervision. A plan of care, signed by a physician, is developed for every patient at the time of admission. This plan is reviewed and revised as needed, based on the patient's/client's health status and at least every 62 days, or according to hospice benefit periods. All interim verbal orders must be promptly confirmed in writing and signed by the physician. All interventions and treatments provided by home care staff are to be consistent with the plan of care. The nurse/therapist is guided by established professional standards in following orders from a physician when any valid question arises. The chair of the professional advisory committee may be consulted when indicated.
- The plan of care uses a standard format that defines the principal diagnoses of the patient and other diagnoses relevant to the care ordered. It must include orders for
    - therapeutic care, activities, diet, and special instructions
    - laboratory tests, X-rays, and the like
    - dosage, frequency, and route of administration of medications
    - treatments requiring the addition of a drug (*Note:* Physician's orders are not required on nonprescription medications when a physician orders a medication through a prescription given either directly to the patient or to the pharmacist. There is no need for contact with the physician unless the nurse has reason to question the use of the medication or has determined that the drug has adversely affected the patient.)
    - supportive care and treatments, including massage, exercise, and safety training by physical, occupational, or speech therapist
    - equipment, supplies, and adaptive devices needed
    - teaching of patient/family indicated by the patient's needs
    - home health aide care
    - precautions and limitations that may affect implementation of the plan

PROCEDURE:

Action	Rationale
1. Demographic and clinical information is obtained when the patient is referred. If the diagnosis is not available, signs and symptoms are recorded and the physician is contacted to obtain diagnosis, prognosis, and additional information.	1. Provision of complete and accurate information to the agency promotes continuity of care and expedites staff assignments and initial assessment.
2. If the patient is receiving care from more than one physician, the nurse is responsible to the referring physician until a coordinated plan can be achieved.	2. Each patient's care must be directed by a primary physician who is aware of all aspects of care.
3. If the referred patient is not under medical supervision, the nurse may make one visit to ascertain needs and assist the patient in obtaining medical supervision from a private physician or hospital clinic.	3. Home care services cannot be initiated without an oral or written plan of care prescribed by physician.

4. Nurse will report complete and accurate clinical information to the physician in accordance with the peer review organization standards.	4. Pennsylvania Keystone Peer Review Organization standards mandate the reporting of a variety of complications and problems to the physician to ensure quality and continuity of care.
5. The primary nurse/therapist who is assigned to the patient makes the initial visit and coordinates the complete plan of treatment with the patient, the physician, and other care providers.	5. A complete, coordinated plan of treatment is better accomplished when one person is assigned overall responsibility. The content of the plan is mandated by Medicare Conditions of Participation.
6. The initial plan of treatment and all interim verbal orders are sent to the physician for signature. The physician is expected to sign and return the orders within 21 to 30 days.	6. Physician signature on all orders is required by law.
7. Signed plans of treatments, certifications, recertifications, and orders changing the plan of treatment (verbal orders) are accepted via fax. A duplicate copy is retained in the office until the original is returned by the physician.	7. Signed fax documents provide for immediate confirmation of orders, when necessary, until signed original is returned to office.
8. If the primary nurse has a question about the validity of any physician's order, he or she should clarify the order with the attending physician, the hospice or medical director, the clinical supervisor, or, if necessary, with the chair of the professional advisory committee before proceeding.	8. Professional nurses carry the ultimate professional responsibility for their individual practice.
9. Physicians who are on the hospital staff are educated on their responsibilities in the management of a home care hospice patient through a letter from the home care executive director. This letter is included in a mailing to all physicians through the chief-of-staff on a periodic basis.	9. This ensures compliance with Joint Commission standards.
10. Physicians who are not on the hospital staff are educated through a letter from the home care executive director that is included with the first medical orders that are mailed for signature.	10. This ensures compliance with Joint Commission standards.

Origin Date: _____
Revised Date: _____
Approved Date: _____
Originator: _____
Distribution: _____

1:44
MEDICATION

PURPOSE:

To establish a policy for the administration of medications to meet the therapeutic needs of the patient consistent with the Medicare Conditions of Participation

RESPONSIBLE PERSONNEL:

Clinical supervisors, registered nurses

OBJECTIVES:

To develop a procedure for the administration, supervision, and instruction of medications

POLICY:

Patients will be instructed on self-administration of medication. In the event that the patient is unable to self-administer or does not possess an understanding of the medication regime, caregivers will be expected to assume this responsibility. When deemed appropriate and when ordered by the physician, nursing staff may administer medications to the patient. Prior to administration, the nurse must review the medication label for the patient's name, drug, dosage, prescription, and expiration date. The nursing staff are generally responsible for the supervision and teaching of medications.

PROCEDURE:

Action

Rationale

Administration

1. Home care staff administer all categories of drugs with the exception of blood products. Examples include the following:
   - bronchodilators by inhalation
   - gold compounds by IM route
   - coagulants and anticoagulants by oral, subcutaneous, IM, and IV routes
   - antibiotics and antifungals by oral, topical, IM, or IV routes (Home care staff may not administer first dose of penicillin or related drugs.)
   - antineoplastic drugs by oral, subcutaenous, IM, or IV routes
   - narcotic analgesics by oral, rectal, subcutaneous, IM, IV, or epidural routes

1. The State Board of Nursing establishes guidelines for the safe practice of nursing in the state. Blood and blood components will not be given by home care staff.

- selected anesthetics for analgesia that may be given via epidural and intrathecal
- other drugs and classes of drugs that may be administered as ordered by attending physician and determined to be safe practice by hospital pharmacy and/or PAC
- diuretics, which may be given IM or IV, including furosemide

2. The hospital pharmacy provides a formulary of drugs categorized by class, and a pharmacist is available by phone to provide information regarding drugs to the home care staff.

3. Drugs may be administered by the home care staff pending verification by physician's order.

2. The hospital pharmacy is a valuable resource in providing guidance in direction regarding administration of drugs.

Supervision and Teaching

1. Nursing staff will check all prescription and nonprescription medications that a patient may be taking to identify:
   - possible ineffective drug therapy (Staff may contact the hospital's drug information center.)
   - adverse reactions (Staff may contact hospital's adverse drug reaction hotline.)
   - drug interactions
   - drug stability (visual review of drug for signs of deterioration, dampness, cloudiness, discoloration, expiration date, storage conditions.)

2. Staff will assess for contraindications based on
   - known drug/food allergies
   - drug incompatibilities, including antagonists
   - patient's/client's physical or mental condition
   - relevant patient/client laboratory results
   - previous reaction to the drug administration

3. The patient/significant others will be instructed in actions, dosage, frequency,

1. Supervision and teaching of medications is standard nursing practice. (*Note:* Physician orders are not required on nonprescription medications or when a physician orders a medication through a prescription given either directly to the patient or to the pharmacist. There is no need for contact with the physician unless the nurse has reason to question the use of the medication or has determined that the drug has adversely affected the patient.)

2. To determine potential food interactions, potential allergic risks, or history of drug interactions and incompatibilities.

3. The goal is independence of patient and family in care.

route, recognition of adverse reactions, and possible drug interactions and appropriate action when adverse drug reaction occurs, as well as in the proper use and maintenance of drug delivery equipment and supplies and the storage and handling of drugs and the delivery system.

4. The patient/significant others will be supervised in medication regimen.

4. The goal is independence of patient and family in care.

Adverse Drug Reactions

1. The physician will be contacted regarding any adverse drug reactions. Staff may consult the adverse drug reaction hotline to address questions concerning adverse drug reactions.

1. Physician must be notified of adverse drug reactions.

2. Significant adverse drug reactions are defined as any situation in which medication elicits specific signs and symptoms of a reaction not directly associated with that medication, such as anaphylaxis, hives/rash, bronchospasm/difficulty in breathing, respiratory depression, gastrointestinal symptoms, cardiovascular symptoms, and central nervous system symptoms. In addition, a significant adverse drug reaction may
    - require discontinuing a medication or modifying the dose
    - require hospitalization
    - result in disability
    - require treatment with a prescription medication
    - result in cognitive impairment
    - result in death or be life threatening
    - result in congenital anomalies

2. Significant adverse drug reactions are reported internally to minimize recurrence and improved performance.

3. Incident reports are the means by which the department identifies and tracks these reactions (Policy 1:32). Adverse drug reactions are tracked and reported annually as part of the program evaluation. The hospital pharmacy is available for consultation and direction on the appropriate external reporting mechanism.

3. All significant adverse reactions are investigated to prevent or reduce the likelihood of such reactions in the future. When deemed appropriate, significant drug reactions will be reported to external sources.

4. In the event of anaphylactic shock, staff will follow the anaphylactic policy and

4. Treatments for adverse reactions are addressed in specific policies. Physicians

comply with emergency procedures.

Medication Errors

1. Medication errors are defined as
   - medications administered by the nurse without an order
   - wrong medication administered by nurse
   - wrong dose or extra dose administered by nurse
   - improper order
   - incorrect mode and time of administration by nurse
   - omission of ordered drug
   - pharmacy dispensing error
   - unprescribed medication taken or medication not taken as prescribed
2. The individual making or discovering the error notifies the supervisor and completes an incident report. Medication errors are tracked and reported annually as part of the annual agency evaluation. The quality improvement process provides a mechanism for addressing unusual trends or incidents.

Unlabeled Drugs

1. Nurses will not assume responsibility for administering or supervising the taking of unlabeled drugs.
2. In the case of an incompletely labeled drug, the nurse will attempt to verify the contents with the physician/pharmacy who dispensed the medication.

Intramuscular/Subcutaneous/Intravenous

1. Nurses may administer injections when physician's order includes name of drug, dosage, frequency, and route.
2. When the nurse notes significant drug reaction in a patient, the physician will be notified and/or the orders for anaphy-

must be notified of any adverse drug reactions.

1. Definition of medication errors is extrapolated from the hospital's incident report document.

2. The quality improvement process provides a mechanism for addressing unusual trends or incidents.

1. To administer unverified unlabeled medication is against the Nurse Practice Act and standards of practice.
2. To administer unverified unlabeled medication is against the Nurse Practice Act and standards of practice.

1. Nurses follow standard nursing practice.

2. Physician is responsible for prescribing medications.

Policies and Procedures

laxis will be followed, depending on the situation.

3. The nurse may teach the patient/significant others to administer injections.

4. The nurse will instruct the patient/significant others in drug actions, dosage, frequency, route, adverse reactions, appropriate action when adverse drug reaction occurs as well as in the proper use and maintenance of drug delivery equipment and supplies, and the storage and handling of drugs and delivery systems.

5. Request for injectable/intravenous medications will be evaluated on an individual basis for safety in the home. Home care supervisors obtain drug information from drug books or by contacting the pharmacy. If there is any question about the safety of the drug, the hospice medical director, a medical representative of the professional advisory committee, and/or the hospital pharmacy will be consulted.

6. Nurse may not administer the first dose of penicillin and derivatives. Nurse may not administer desensitizing drugs.

7. Nursing staff will adhere to the following protocol for intramuscular administration of Imferon:
   - Do not administer the initial dose of Imferon.
   - Position patient in prone position (recommended).
   - Administer deep into upper outer quadrant of the gluteus maximus.
   - Use needle at least two inches long (gauge #19 or #20).
   - Introduce a small amount of air into syringe after measuring drug.
   - Retract skin laterally before inserting needle (z track technique).

8. Nursing personnel may administer intramuscular Solganal for its anti-inflammatory effects in the treatment of rheumatoid arthritis. Patient must be under close medical supervision. Monitoring for hematologic dyscrasia should be done

---

3. The goal is independence of patient and family in care.

4. Safety and infection control are ensured.

5. Patient safety is ensured.

6. The medication must be administered under medical direction where emergency measures can be initiated in case of adverse reactions.

7. Agency follows *Physicians Desk Reference* recommendations for administration of Imferon.
   - Risk of anaphylaxis

   - Risk of staining skin, necrosis, atrophy, fibrosis
   - As above

   - As above

   - Clean needle of medicine post injection
   - Risk of staining skin, necrosis, atrophy, fibrosis

8. Agency follows *Physicians Desk Reference* recommendations for administration of Solganal.

every two to four weeks; urinalysis for protein levels should be performed weekly prior to the weekly gold administration or as per physician's orders. Toxic signs and symptoms usually occur when the patient has received 250–500 mgm cumulative of the gold salt and include urticaria, dermatitis, stomatitis, vaginitis, etc. Nursing staff will adhere to the following protocol for the administration of Solganal:

- Immerse in warm H_2O and shake vial thoroughly.
- Position patient in prone position (recommended).
- Use needle at least 1-1/2–2 inches long (gauge #18).

- Administer deep into upper quadrant of the gluteus maximus.
- Observe patient for approximately 15 minutes post injection.

- Must warm and shake the Solganal suspension vigorously
- To minimize adverse effects of hypotension
- To prevent localized skin reaction, as dermatitis is the most common adverse reaction of the drug
- As above

- Risk of anaphylaxis

IV Administration of Furosemide

1. Nursing staff may administer IV furosemide (Lasix). It is recommended that the nurse administer no more than 80 mg at one time every 12 hours to a maximum of 160 mg per day. However, the dosage may be altered at the discretion of the physician. The medication must be administered slowly over one to two minutes. When receiving this therapy, the patient must be under close medical supervision. Monitoring for electrolyte imbalance should be done weekly or as per physician's order. The order for IV Lasix may be renewed at the discretion of the physician but not less than once every 62 days.

1. Agency follows *Physicians Desk Reference* recommendations for administration of IV Lasix. Protocol is in compliance with professional advisory committee recommendation.

Drugs Given for Research Purposes

1. Nurses may administer codified or experimental drugs under the following conditions:

1. This policy was developed for the protection of patients and nursing staff.

- If hospice IDG and professional advisory approval has been obtained
- If the written order includes content of preparation, therapeutic effect expected, untoward or unfavorable reactions, and symptoms to report to physician
- If the order is given by a physician associated with a reputable institution involved in research
- If the container is properly marked with the same code number that is written on the order sheet
- If the home care agency has a photocopy of consent form signed by the patient in the hospital

Before administering codified medications, the nurse must be aware of all potential untoward reactions and side effects and the therapeutic effects to be anticipated. It is also important that patients understand the treatment and possible side effects.

Origin Date: _____
Revised Date: _____
Approved Date: _____
Originator: _____
Distribution: _____

1:45
NURSING SERVICES

PURPOSE:

To provide a description of the scope of practice for skilled nursing services in the home care program

RESPONSIBLE PERSONNEL:

Professional advisory committee, executive director, director of professional services, registered nurses

OBJECTIVES:

- To provide a physician, nursing, psychosocial, safety and environmental assessment
- To establish a description and criteria for skilled nursing services
- To provide nursing services to patients with the goal of encouraging and assisting patients and families to achieve the maximum degree of independence possible

- To provide optimal care to patients in accordance with the state's Nurse Practice Act and established professional nursing standards

POLICY:

- Skilled nursing services are provided to patients in their homes or in other appropriate settings, with the frequency and pattern of visiting based on patient/family needs and patient service priorities. Nursing services include:
  - Assessment of physical, nursing, psychosocial, spiritual, and environmental needs of the patient/family.
  - Collaboration with the attending physician and hospice IDG in establishing a treatment plan.
  - Provision and demonstration of nursing procedures, techniques, skills. In the absence of specific orders, the nurse will comply with stated nursing procedures and standing orders as stated in nursing procedure manual.
  - Teaching and counseling for health promotion/prevention.
  - Identifying the need for other agency or community services and initiating the appropriate referrals.
  - Promotion of continuity of care through coordination of patient care services.
  - Ongoing evaluation of the patient/family response to nursing care.
  - Direction and supervision of home health aide or a substitute family member in the provision of patient care.
- All therapeutic services are provided with close communication and cooperation of the medical profession, with an accompanying physician's plan of care in writing, signed by the physician. The scope of nursing practice is defined by the Nurse Practice Act of the state. Nursing is defined as the diagnosis and treatment of human responses to actual or potential health problems. The "practice of professional nursing" means diagnosing and treating human responses to actual or potential health problems through such services as case finding, health teaching, health counseling, provision of care supportive to or restorative of life and well-being, and executing medical regimens as prescribed by a licensed physician or dentist (Penn. Act No. 69, Section 2 (1), the Professional Nursing Law, of 1951 and subsequent amendments).

PROCEDURE:

Skilled professional nursing is provided by a licensed registered nurse (refer to job description for position qualification) in accordance with the plan of care prescribed by a physician. Nurses carry out the following functions:

Action	Rationale
Patient Care	
1. Make an initial patient evaluation visit on all referred patients, initiate or complete the plan of care, communicate the	1. This and all the following patient care measures constitute the scope of nursing practice in a home care/hospice setting.

evaluation of the patient's condition to the physician and the hospice IDG.
2. Reassess the patient's condition and inform the physician and other members of the interdisciplinary team of changes on each visit. For patients receiving care on an inpatient level, daily patient reassessment responsibilities will be delegated to an inpatient facility staff. These assessments will be monitored and evaluated by the hospice staff.
3. Provide those services prescribed on the plan of care that require substantial and specialized nursing skill.
4. Initiate appropriate therapeutic nursing measures.
5. Counsel the patient and family in meeting the nursing and health care needs of the patient.
6. Serve as primary clinician, when so assigned, coordinating care and initiating team conferences as indicated by the patient's needs.
7. Initiates 62-day written summary (or according to hospice benefit periods) of the patient's care and response for the patient's attending physician and the physician's recertification of plan of care.
8. Prepare a discharge summary at the termination of care.
9. Prepare clinical and progress notes on every patient contact according to establish policy. (Refer to Policy 1:10, Clinical Records.)

Other Functions

1. Supervise the care given by the home health aide/homemaker to patients for whom the home health nurse is the primary clinician. A supervisory visit is made every two weeks and documented on the record.
2. Coordinate with other professional disciplines in the home health/hospice program to provide comprehensive services to assigned patients.

1. The nurse is responsible for supervising nursing care delegated to paraprofessionals.

2. The assigned primary nurse is responsible for coordination of the care planning and services rendered to the patient.

3. Assist in orientation of home health nurses as assigned.

4. Participate in staff development opportunities according to the identified needs of the individual and the organization.

3. Experienced nurses act as mentors of new nurses, demonstrating needed skills and sharing knowledge.

4. Participation in staff development activities keeps nurses current with needs in home care.

Services Not Permitted

1. Nurses may not administer the first dose of penicillin and derivatives.

1. The medications must be administered under medical direction where emergency measures can be instituted in case of adverse reactions.

2. Nurses may not administer desensitizing drugs.

Origin Date: _____
Revised Date: _____
Approved Date: _____
Originator: _____
Distribution: _____

1:46
OCCUPATIONAL THERAPY SERVICES

PURPOSE:

To provide a description of the scope of practice of the occupational therapy services in the home care/hospice program (in accordance with the Pennsylvania Standards of Practice)

RESPONSIBLE PERSONNEL:

Director of professional services, therapy supervisor, hospice coordinator, occupational therapists

OBJECTIVES:

- To evaluate patient's home setting
- To assess patient's physical/mental and functional limitations and assets
- To promote community understanding of occupational therapy services
- To assist in the coordination of activities with other personnel and other community agencies in bringing about such physical, psychological, social, economic, and vocational adjustments as may be indicated in the best interest of the patient
- To provide continuity of care to patients recently discharged from the hospital after receiving services
- To assist the patients in adjustment to the illness by
  - assisting patients in planning modifications in their surroundings and in achieving maximum physical independence
  - providing assistance to the family in the adjustment to the disability
- To delineate qualifications of the occupational therapist responsible for the provision of care (refer to job description)

POLICY:

- Occupational therapy is a patient care service that provides care to persons who have acute conditions, short-term illnesses, long-term disabilities, or terminal illness. Qualified therapists work as members of the home care/hospice team in a community setting and provide service to patients based on the referral and written prescription of a physician.
- The professional practice of occupational therapy is directed toward the following:
  - Assessment of physical abilities, disabilities, and limitations and of architectural and environmental barriers
  - Relieving pain
  - Preventing further deformity
  - Developing or improving activities of daily living
- Maintaining maximum performance within the patient's capabilities. Such direction is executed by using such evaluative procedures as manual muscle examinations, functional evaluations, sensory testing, measurements of range of motion, assessment of cognitive/perceptual testing development and utilization of human movement, and activities of daily living. Physical therapeutic agents, such as the application of heat, cold, water, massage, and various assistive devices, are also used to assist the patient toward a rehabilitative goal.
- Occupational therapy services are provided to patients who are currently under the care of a physician and receiving skilled nursing, physical therapy, or speech therapy.

PROCEDURE:

Action	Rationale
Occupational therapy services are provided by qualified occupational therapists in accordance with a plan of treatment prescribed by a physician. Therapists carry out the following functions.	These measures constitute the scope of occupational therapy practice in a home care setting and comply with Medicare Conditions of Participation.

Direct Service

1. Provide an assessment of the patient's abilities, disabilities, and limitations and develop the plan of care within five days.
2. Provide occupational therapy for hospice patients who are in an environment where treatment goals may be continued and reinforced.
3. Perform selected procedures as ordered by the physician and as warranted by the patient's clinical status.

4. Teach selected procedures as ordered by the physician and as warranted by the patient's clinical status.
5. Provide written instructions to patients for activities to be carried out between visits.
6. Assess total patient and family needs and, when necessary, make referrals to available community resources to meet these needs.

Consultation Service

1. Provide office consultation to the nurse and hospice IDG and, when necessary, make joint field visits to coordinate occupational therapy service for newly admitted patients or patients for whom planned nursing and occupational therapy have already been established.

Supervision of Aides

1. Provide a written outline of the occupational therapy procedures to the home health aide and demonstrate the procedures to the aide.
2. Refer the patient requiring home health aide service for occupational therapy to the nurse who supervises the aide. The nurse makes supervisory visits every two weeks to observe the patient and the home health aide's functioning.

Documentation

1. Request the initial occupational therapy orders from the physician.
2. Review the plan of care with the hospice IDG, and renew the plan of treatment with the physician every 62 days, or according to hospice benefit periods.
3. Obtain verbal orders as indicated by the patient's changing status. (Refer to Policy 1:43, Medical Services.)

4. Complete an assessment and plan of care within five days.
5. Revise the plan as needed. Incorporate revisions in the clinical note.
6. Reassess the patient's status and progress on each visit, documenting in the clinical note. Complete a new evaluation and plan of care form after each hospitalization.
7. Keep complete and accurate records on all patients receiving occupational therapy service by completing a clinical note on every visit.
8. Record on the patient record all field consultation and evaluation service.
9. Provide all pertinent communications pertaining to patient's care, progress, and status to the appropriate persons.
10. Conference with nurses/other hospice disciplines.
11. Complete physician's plan of treatment on admission and every 62 days thereafter, or according to hospice benefit periods.
12. Complete verbal orders as needed.

Origin Date: _____
Revised Date: _____
Approved Date: _____
Originator: _____
Distribution: _____

1:47
OPERATIONAL AGREEMENT WITH PASTORAL CARE

PURPOSE:

To provide a clinical facility for hospital chaplaincy residents to help meet the spiritual needs of clients in the home

RESPONSIBLE PERSONNEL:

Hospital chaplains, AMHHC hospice chaplain, AMHHC hospice supervisor, AMHHC volunteer director (bereavement), and clinical educator

POLICY:

Clinical experience is available to meet the needs of patients, residents, and staff, subject to procedures listed below

PROCEDURE:

Action	Rationale
1. The number of residents sent to AMHHC by pastoral care shall not exceed one at any one time.	1. This is the maximum number of residents that can be accommodated by the staff.
2. The AMHHC will provide each resident with orientation and observation under the direction of the hospice team and/or clinical educator.	2. The professional staff serve as a role model for residents.
3. Pastoral care will provide the AMHHC with a master schedule listing names of residents and dates of the planned experience prior to beginning of experience. In the event of any change in schedules, either party may notify the other of the change either orally or in writing.	3. The advance notice allows time for the staff to schedule resident visits.
4. Pastoral care agrees to have its residents: • Abide by general policies of the AMHHC when visiting patients, as directed by staff, when observing or when visiting individually • Keep confidential all knowledge and records of patients • Visit only those patients who are currently receiving AMHHC services	• The care of the patient is foremost. • This meets certification, accreditation, and professional standards. • This complies with hospital policies/procedures.
5. AMHHC will make available to residents all pertinent educational material during period of observation.	5. The AMHHC is a partner in the educational process.
6. In the event of accident, injury, or illness of resident on observation experience, AMHHC will notify pastoral care, and plans for residents return to hospital will be made on an individual basis, dependent on situation. Pastoral care shall assume responsibility for care and emergency transportation of resident.	6. This meets hospital's policies/procedures.
7. The faculty of the pastoral care department agrees to present the terminal evaluation of the observation experience to the executive director of AMHHC within 30 days of its completion.	7. The evaluations by residents are included as one aspect of the total annual agency evaluation process.
8. Pastoral care residents will provide individual malpractice insurance coverage.	8. This meets hospital requirements.

Origin Date: _____

Revised Date: _____

Approved Date: _____

Originator: _____

Distribution: _____

Policies and Procedures 107

1:48
ORGANIZATIONAL CHART
ABINGTON MEMORIAL HOSPITAL HOME CARE HOSPICE PROGRAM

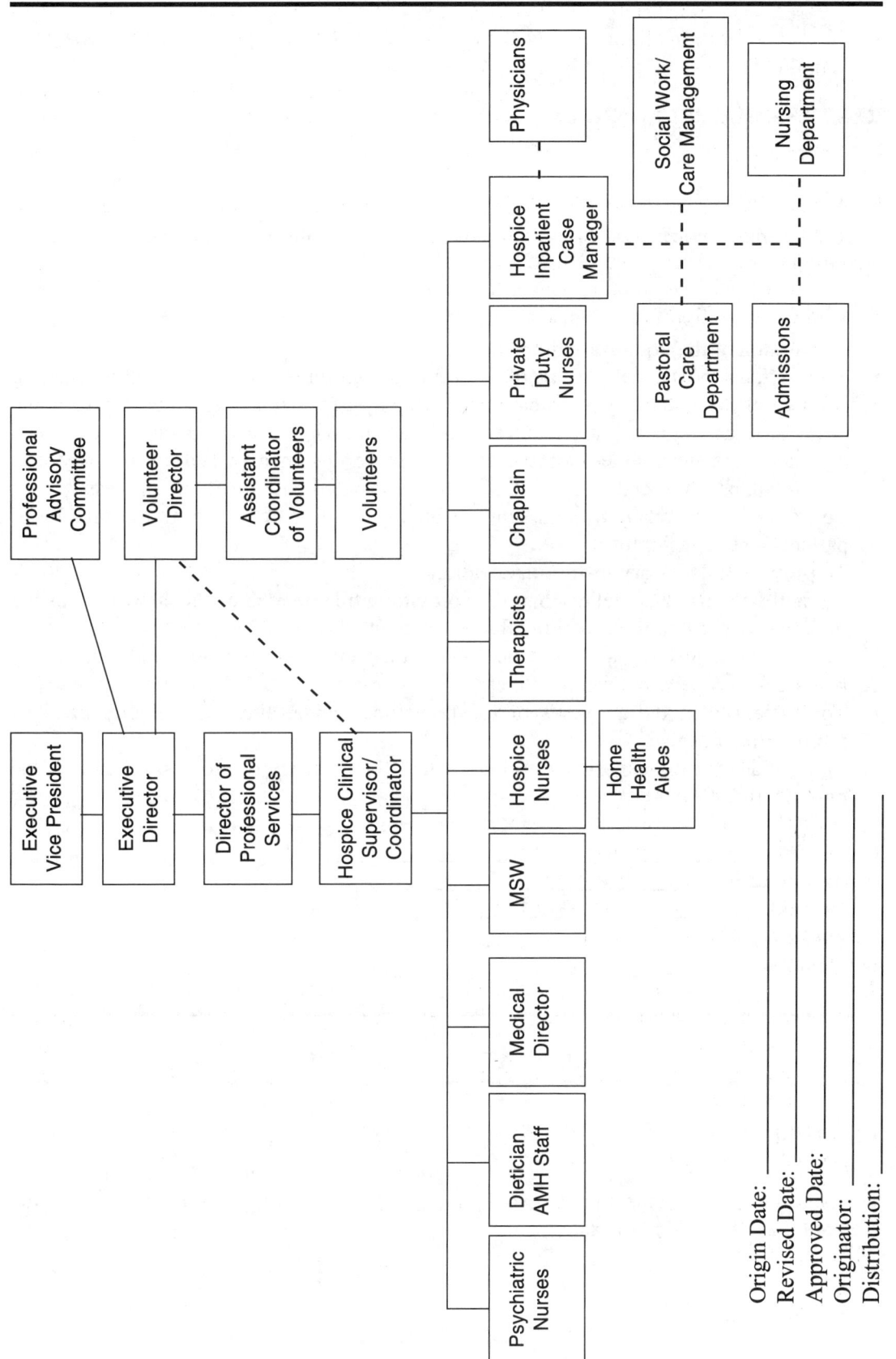

Origin Date: _____
Revised Date: _____
Approved Date: _____
Originator: _____
Distribution: _____

1:49
ORGANIZATIONAL MISSION

PURPOSE:

To define the mission for which the organization exists

RESPONSIBLE PERSONNEL:

Governing body

OBJECTIVES:

To define the organizational mission that governs the scope and practices of the organization's operations

POLICY:

The mission of the organization is:
- To provide professional and ancillary services including, but not limited to, nursing service, physical therapy, occupational therapy, speech therapy, social work, home health aide, chaplain, volunteer, and counseling to individuals in their place of residence, or other locations deemed appropriate, which are designed to address the physical, emotional, psychosocial, and spiritual issues associated with the dying process
- To promote comprehensive and superior quality health care services to terminally ill patients and their families
- To prevent unnecessary institutionalization
- To facilitate early hospital discharge by providing treatment that is technically feasible in the residence and most beneficial to the patient
- To provide counseling and guidance in locating and using personal and community resources to cope with terminal illness
- To participate in the activities of local, regional, state, and national organizations representing hospice
- To provide learning experiences for students from a variety of professions and for the community at large

Origin Date: _____
Revised Date: _____
Approved Date: _____
Originator: _____
Distribution: _____

1:50
ORIENTATION/EDUCATION

PURPOSE:

To provide a written plan for the orientation of new personnel (including contract personnel) to the concepts and philosophy unique to hospice care and to provide ongoing education as deemed appropriate

RESPONSIBLE PERSONNEL:

The hospice interdisciplinary group

OBJECTIVES:

- To promote understanding of the origin and philosophy of the hospice program
- To orient personnel to charting and communication requirements
- To provide inservice training to staff and contract personnel
- To educate staff on the importance of the coordination of activities and services provided by staff and contract personnel

POLICY:

- The agency assumes responsibility for orientation and continuing education of all hospice personnel, including contract personnel.
- Orientation specific to the hospice program is conducted by the hospice coordinator (or designee) in conjunction with the hospice team. This orientation is completed prior to the initiation of service to hospice benefit patients.
- Programs suitable for the continuing education of hospice team members will be available through the staff development program of AMHHC. Continuing education programs are offered in consultation with the medical director.
- The hospice coordinator or designee will also provide continuing education to all members of the hospice team, including contract personnel, on issues specific to hospice as those needs are identified.

PROCEDURE:

Action	Rationale
1. The governing body and administration will provide the framework, staff, and funds to facilitate an ongoing program.	1. The hospice retains responsibility for appropriate hospice care training of personnel.
2. All staff and contractors complete orientation specific to hospice prior to their initiation of hospice services.	2. Orientation for newly appointed members of the staff/contractors will facilitate their understanding of their responsibilities and the hospice program.
3. Based on the needs of the staff/contractors and the organization, educational programs are made available.	3. There is opportunity for learning experiences to occur within the agency as well as off-site.
4. The hospice makes journals and educational materials available to staff/contractors.	4. Staff/contractors have the opportunity to access information for the purpose of self-enrichment.

Origin Date: _____
Revised Date: _____
Approved Date: _____
Originator: _____
Distribution: _____

1:51
PAIN AND SYMPTOM MANAGEMENT

POLICY:

- The hospice program provides assistance to patient/family in pain and symptom management in cooperation with the patient's physician.
- Pain and symptom management is based on the assessment of the primary nurse and the needs of the patient. The interdisciplinary team communicates and consults with the attending physician regarding the results of symptom control. Patients and families are instructed in necessary measures to provide safe symptom management in the absence of the nurse. Frequent reassessment of the patient's symptoms will be done by the professional staff and communicated by the team members at team conference. The pain assessment form is to be used as an option for difficult pain management (Form 24).
- Twenty-four hour pharmacy calls are taken by contract pharmacy.
- Twenty-four hour pharmacy calls for intravenous needs will be handled by contracted pharmacy. Twenty-four hour pharmacy and intravenous needs for patients hospitalized for acute inpatient care will be managed by Abington Memorial Hospital staff.

Origin Date: _____
Revised Date: _____
Approved Date: _____
Originator: _____
Distribution: _____

1:52
PATIENT'S BILL OF RIGHTS/RESPONSIBILITIES

PURPOSE:

To provide information to patients that describes their rights and responsibilities related to their care and how to communicate comments to administration

RESPONSIBLE PERSONNEL:

Executive director, director of professional services, visiting staff, legal counsel

OBJECTIVES:

- To inform the patient that he or she has the right:
  - To make informed decisions regarding care
  - To receive needed care in a timely and competent manner
  - To voice grievances and recommend change in policies and service without coercion, discrimination, refusal, or unreasonable interruption of service
  - To assure patients that information related to them is confidential

POLICY:

Each patient will receive a copy of the Patient's Bill of Rights and Responsibilities on admission for home care services prior to the provision of service.

PROCEDURE:

Action

1. On admission, each patient is given a copy out of the Patient's Bill of Rights and Responsibilities.
2. The staff member reviews the document with the patient/family as part of the admissions procedure prior to the provision of service.
3. The patient and witness sign and date the form. One copy is left with the patient. The second copy is filed in the clinical record.

Rationale

1. To meet agency policy and Medicare requirements.
2. To ensure that all patients understand the contents of the document.
3. To document that information and required materials have been given to patient.

Origin Date: _____
Revised Date: _____
Approved Date: _____
Originator: _____
Distribution: _____

1:53
PHYLSICAL THERAPY SERVICES

PURPOSE:

To provide a description of the scope of practice of the physical therapy services in the home care/hospice program (in accordance with the Pennsylvania Standards of Practice)

RESPONSIBLE PERSONNEL:

Director of professional services, therapy supervisor, hospice coordinator, physical therapists

OBJECTIVES:

- To assess the patient's ability, disability, and limitations
- To assist patients in adjustment to the disease process by:
  - assisting patients in planning modifications to their surroundings and in achieving maximum functional abilities
  - providing assistance to the family in the adjustment to the disease process
- To assist in the coordination of activities with agency personnel and other community agencies in bringing about such physical, psychological, social, economic, and vocational adjustments as may be indicated in the best interest of the patient
- To promote community understanding of physical therapy services
- To delineate qualifications of the physical therapist responsible for the provision of care (see job description)

POLICY:

- Physical therapy is a patient care service that provides care to persons who have acute conditions, short-term illnesses, long-term disabilities, or terminal illness. Qualified physical therapists work as members of the home care/hospice team in a community setting and provide service to patients based on the referral and written prescription of a physician.
- The professional practice of physical therapy is directed toward:
  - Assessment of physical abilities, disabilities, and limitations and of architectural/environmental barriers and psychosocial status.
  - Relieving pain.
  - Preventing further deformity.
  - Developing or improving body skills.
  - Maintaining maximum performance within the patient's capabilities. Such direction is executed by using evaluative procedures such as manual and electrical muscle examinations, functional evaluations, gait analysis, sensory testing, measurements of range of motion, and assessment of development and utilization of human movement. Physical therapeutic agents, such as the application of heat, cold, water, electricity, massage, and various supportive devices, are also used to assist the patient toward a rehabilitative goal.

PROCEDURE:

Action

Physical therapy services are provided by licensed physical therapists in accordance with the physical therapy standards of practice and the plan of care prescribed by a physician. Therapists carry out the following functions.

Rationale

These measures constitute the scope of physical therapy practice in a home care setting and comply with Medicare Conditions of Participation.

Direct Service

1. Provide an assessment of the patient's abilities, disabilities, and limitations.
2. Develop a plan of care based on the assessment within five days.
3. Provide physical therapy for hospice patients.
4. Provide physical therapy services to patients on an outpatient basis.
5. Perform selected procedures as ordered by the physician and as warranted by the patient's clinical status.
6. Teach selected procedures to a responsible member of the family.

7. Provide written instructions to patients for activities to be carried out between visits.
8. Assess total patient and family needs and, when necessary, make referrals to available community resources to meet those needs.

Consultation Service

1. Provide office consultation to the nurse or hospice IDG, and make field visits to coordinate physical therapy service for newly admitted patients or those for whom planned nursing and physical therapy has already been established.

Supervision of Aides

1. Provide a written outline of the procedures to the home health aide and demonstrate the procedures to the aide. File a copy in the patient's record and forward a copy to the home health aide supervisor.
2. Provide supervision every two weeks to the home health aide to observe the home health aide's demonstration of the procedures and to make any indicated changes.

Documentation

1. Request the initial physical therapy orders from the physician.
2. Review the plan of care with the hospice IDG and renew the plan of treatment with the physician every 62 days, or per hospice benefit period.
3. Obtain verbal orders as indicated by patient's changing status. (Refer to Policy 1:43, Medical Services.)
4. Complete the assessment and develop the plan of care within five days. Complete a new evaluation and plan of care form after each hospitalization.

5. Revise the plan as needed. Incorporate revision in the clinical note.
6. Reassess the patient's status and progress on each visit, documenting in the clinical note.
7. Keep complete and accurate records on all patients receiving physical therapy service by completing a clinical note on every visit.
8. Record on the patient record all field consultation and evaluation service.
9. Provide all pertinent communications pertaining to patient's care, progress, and status to the appropriate persons.
10. Conference with nurses/other hospice disciplines.
11. Complete physician's plan of treatment on admission and every 62 days thereafter, or according to hospice benefit periods.
12. Complete verbal orders as needed.

Origin Date: _____
Revised Date: _____
Approved Date: _____
Originator: _____
Distribution: _____

1:54
PROGRAM STATEMENT

- The hospice program plays an important role in the community in that it makes available to residents of AMHHC service area a program that allows for care of the terminally ill patient in the home.
- For those patients who are eligible and elect Medicare hospice benefits, Medical Assistance, or other third party, additional services are available as specified by the benefit plan. These may include short-term inpatient care, medical appliances and supplies, drugs and biologicals, continuous care in periods of temporary crisis and short-term respite care.
- In the event that the patient does not elect the hospice benefit, and/or the patient is not eligible for a hospice benefit, the hospice strives to provide the patient with optimal home health services.

Origin Date: _____
Revised Date: _____
Approved Date: _____
Originator: _____
Distribution: _____

1:55
PROTOCOL FOR REFERRALS BETWEEN HOSPITAL AND HOSPICE PROGRAM

PURPOSE:

To promote smooth transition of care between the hospital acute care unit and the home for terminally ill patients and their families

PROCEDURE:

Action	Rationale
1. Case manager identifies patient appropriate for hospice program involvement. • Complete assessment form. • Confirm patient/family awareness of diagnosis/prognosis. • Secure prognosis from physician to ensure appropriateness for hospice. • Confirm social service involvement. • Assess patient for high-tech needs and proceed accordingly. Call information to AMHHC hospice or other appropriate hospice program. • Hospice representative to make inpatient visit if appropriate.	1. These actions provide for a smooth transfer of patient care from the hospital to a home care hospice program.
2. Hospice coordinator will coordinate assignment of primary nurse and team with area nursing supervisor. • Assign nursing assessment according to home care policy. • Notify team by phone or call team meeting, if appropriate. • Confirm any applicable hospice benefits via AMHHC business office. • Ensure that informed consent for hospice benefit patients are secured by home care staff.	2. These actions provide for continuity of patient care.
3. AMHHC hospice patient hospitalized at AMH for inpatient services. • Hospice coordinator to notify appropriate team members of patient admission to AMH. • Hospice coordinator or designee will provide appropriate orientation to inpatient staff.	3. These actions provide for a smooth transfer of patient care from the home to the inpatient hospice unit.

- Inpatient hospice case manager or designee will establish and deliver plan of care to nursing station for inclusion on AMH chart.
- Inpatient hospice case manager or designee will be in contact with patient and inpatient facility on regular basis to manage further developments in plan of care for Medicare benefit patients.
- Inpatient hospice case manager or designee will coordinate discharge planning needs for patients resuming home services.

Origin Date: _____
Revised Date: _____
Approved Date: _____
Originator: _____
Distribution: _____

1:56
PURPOSE AND GOALS OF HOSPICE PROGRAM

- The AMHHC hospice program was developed for the purpose of providing palliative supportive home care services to patients with a terminal illness. The hospice program interdisciplinary group consists of a medical director, professional nurses, medical social workers, coordinator of volunteers, chaplain, and volunteers. Additional support for the individual patient may include home health aides, homemakers, physical therapists, occupational therapists, speech pathologists, and registered dietitians. The focus of the interdisciplinary group is the provision of comprehensive home care services to the dying patient and his or her family. Following the death of the patient, the surviving family is eligible for bereavement counseling support for up to one year.
- The goals of the hospice program are to allow a patient to live out his or her days in an environment of choice, be surrounded by familiar persons, be free of pain, live with mental alertness, and have professional help in coping with the physical and emotional stresses associated with the dying process.

Origin Date: _____
Revised Date: _____
Approved Date: _____
Originator: _____
Distribution: _____

1:57
QUALITY ASSESSMENT AND IMPROVEMENT PROGRAM

POLICY:

The hospice program strives to ensure the provision of high-quality patient/family care through an ongoing comprehensive assessment of the quality and appropriateness of care. A quality assessment and improvement team, consisting of the quality assessment and improvement (QAI) supervisor, the hospice coordinator, and select members of the IDG, maintains responsibility for the hospice QAI program. The QAI supervisor is ultimately responsible for the program. The team reports findings to the administrative staff. The reports are relayed to the board of directors and to the professional advisory committee on a quarterly basis.

OBJECTIVES:

- Patient care will be monitored for the quality and appropriateness of services on a quarterly basis through analysis of patient records, patient questionnaires, and physician questionnaires.
- The IDG will address and resolve identified problems at the weekly meeting or as needed.
- The IDG will make suggestions for improving patient care at the weekly meeting or as needed.

METHODS:

1. *Program Evaluation:* The IDG shall, under the guidance of the hospice coordinator, evaluate selected program issues on a continuing basis. Issues appropriate for ongoing analysis include symptom management, inpatient care, communications, statistical issues, trends of care needs, beeper calls, and so forth. Important aspects of hospice care are incorporated in the AMH home care quality assessment and improvement program.
2. *Quarterly Record Review:* At least 10 percent of hospice patients will be reviewed as part of the quarterly record review program. In addition, hospice benefit patients' charts will be reviewed during the quarterly record review process, to a maximum of 50 records per quarter.
3. *Semiannual Questionnaire:* Hospice patient's survivors receive a follow-up questionnaire eight weeks after the patient's death. Results of the questionnaire survey are analyzed and reported by the QAI supervisor semiannually. Returned questionnaires are also reviewed by team members.
4. *Patient Letters:* Unsolicited patient/family letters are included in the QAI program.
5. *Annual Physician Questionnaires:* All physicians of hospice patients receive questionnaires.
6. *Utilization Review:* Utilization review will be done on all hospice patients evaluated by the quarterly review process.
7. *Annual Agency Evaluation:* At the direction of the executive director, an annual hospice program report will be submitted by the hospice coordinator as part of the annual agency evaluation.

These program issues are considered by the IDG and presented to AMHHC administration by the hospice coordinator or designee and other team members, as appropriate.

The results of the continuing program evaluations and plans are incorporated into the monthly hospice report to hospital administration, which reports to the board of trustees.

Origin Date: _____
Revised Date: _____
Approved Date: _____
Originator: _____
Distribution: _____

1:58
QUARTERLY RECORD REVIEW

OBJECTIVE:

To establish criteria for the assessment of services provided to substantiate adherence to agency policies for maintenance of optimal care, safety, and adequate support services.

METHOD:

1. Quantitative and qualitative review is performed on an approved percentage of randomly selected open and closed records for each discipline on a quarterly basis.
   - The computer system generates a quarterly summary report that provides a numerical list of individuals serviced by all disciplines during the quarter. Based on these data, 10 percent of the records (7 percent if caseload is greater than 500) to a maximum of 50 per discipline per quarter are chosen. If the number is less than 10 cases per discipline for the quarter, all records for that discipline will be reviewed.
   - Records for review may be selected from the quality assessment/performance improvement review list. The visit register and/or the active and discharged chart files may also be used in the selection process.
   - The hospice coordinator will notify the quality assessment supervisor of all hospice patients each quarter. At least 10 percent of hospice records will be included in the AMHHC quality assessment program.
   - For hospice benefit patients receiving inpatient care, either acute or respite care, patient records will be reviewed for quality assessment by the hospice coordinator or designee, to a maximum number of 50 inpatients per quarter.
2. Individual record findings and recommendations are recorded on quality assessment forms.
3. Findings and recommendations are summarized.
4. Summarized findings and recommendations are recorded in
   - committee quarterly minutes and PAC minutes
   - annual report to board of directors at end of fourth quarter as part of agency's program evaluation
5. Summarized findings are presented to staff members to:
   - Identify areas of strengths and weaknesses.
   - Recommend and initiate action for the enhancement of care.
6. In addition to the AMHHC quality assurance program, the following review mechanisms will be employed for hospice patients:
   - The interdisciplinary group conference reviews and revises the plan of care at least biweekly.
   - For patients who receive inpatient care, the hospice coordinator or designee will contact on a regular basis to review the inpatient care and update the plan of care, when indicated.

Origin Date: _____
Revised Date: _____
Approved Date: _____
Originator: _____
Distribution: _____

1:59
RELEASE OF INFORMATION FROM RECORDS CONTAINING HIV-RELATED INFORMATION

PURPOSE:

To establish uniform policy on release of information from patient records covered by Pennsylvania Act 148, the Confidentiality of HIV-Related Information Act of 1990

POLICY:

- The term *HIV-related information* refers to

    any information which is in the possession of a person who provides one or more health or social services or who obtains the information pursuant to a release of confidential HIV-related information and which concerns whether an individual has been the subject of an HIV-related test, or has HIV, HIV-related illness or AIDS; or any information which identifies or reasonably could identify an individual as having one or more of these conditions, including information pertaining to the individual's contacts (Act 148).

- Medical records of all patients undergoing HIV-related testing for diagnostic purposes, medical records of patients tested following an employee's significant exposure, medical records of patients with a diagnosis of AIDS or other recognized HIV-related diagnosis who have not undergone HIV-related testing or treatment during the current admission where HIV-related information is documented, and medical records of all patients with primary or secondary diagnoses of AIDS or HIV-related conditions shall be carefully examined for the presence of HIV-related information and protected by the state regulation.

- Without specific written consent, disclosure of confidential HIV-related information gathered in the course of providing any health or social service is prohibited except if the information is to be released to
    - the patient
    - the physician who ordered the test or his or her designee
    - any person specifically designated in a written consent
    - an agent, employee, or medical staff member of the hospital who is actively engaged in providing treatment for the patient or to those persons at other facilities to which the patient is being transferred and a summary or portion of the record is necessary to provide for continuity of care
    - those participating in a peer review organization or any federal or state government agency with oversight responsibilities with other hospitals, such as Joint Commission or state licensure reviewers and inspectors
    - medical personnel in response to emergency medical situations when release of HIV-related information is necessary to provide care or treatment, in which case only specific information necessary for medical management of the emergency may be released on a nonconsensual basis
    - third-party payers, to the extent necessary to reimburse the hospital or make payment
    - the department of health and persons authorized to gather vital statistics
    - local health boards and departments as authorized by the Disease Prevention and Control Law of 1955

- a person allowed access to the information by court order
- a funeral director responsible for the acceptance and preparation of the deceased patient
- specified county employees
- To disclose information upon a written consent, the authorization must contain the following elements:
  - identity of the patient
  - a time limit on its validity, not to exceed 90 days, which shows starting and ending dates and the event or condition upon which the consent will expire
  - identity of person to whom the records are to be released
  - a statement of the purpose for which the released records are to be used
  - a statement identifying what portions of the records are to be released
  - a place for the signature of the patient/legal guardian, and an area for the date
  - the specific name of the person permitted to make the disclosure
  - indication that the release may be revoked at any time in writing, except to the extent that action has been taken in reliance thereon
  - signature of patient and date authorization was signed
- To prohibit redisclosure of released records, the following statement shall accompany the records:

   This information has been disclosed to you from records protected by Pennsylvania law. Pennsylvania law prohibits you from making any further disclosure of this information unless further disclosure is expressly permitted by the written consent of the person to whom it pertains or is authorized by the confidentiality of HIV-Related Information Act. A general authorization for the release of medical or other information is not sufficient for this purpose.

Origin Date: _____
Revised Date: _____
Approved Date: _____
Originator: _____
Distribution: _____

1:60
SAFETY MANAGEMENT

PURPOSE:

To establish standards to ensure patient and staff safety and minimize hazards related to the provision of care

RESPONSIBLE PERSONNEL:

Executive director, director of professional services, all staff

OBJECTIVES:

- To establish standards to ensure patient and staff safety and to minimize hazards related to the provision of care
- To educate staff and patients to carry out the safety standards, which include but are not limited to

- basic home safety
- safe and appropriate use of equipment
- storage, handling, and delivery of medical equipment and supplies

POLICY:

The home care program has developed basic home safety standards in accordance with the guidelines established by the Department of Health and Human Services and the Consumer Product Safety Commission. In addition, guidelines for medical equipment and supplies have been developed. All staff are oriented to the guidelines upon employment during orientation. Annually, a safety management inservice is held for all employees. Patients and caregivers are given a copy of the home safety standards and instructed in appropriate safety measures specific to their needs. Any incidents are reported according to Policy 1:32.

PROCEDURE:

Action	Rationale
1. The quality assessment/improvement staff development supervisor arranges for all new employees to attend the safety/fire management seminar at the hospital.	1. All employees are thus educated to the established safety guidelines.
2. The home care staff are additionally oriented to the basic home safety standards and the safety guidelines for medical equipment and supplies.	2. These guidelines are followed on all home visits and must be familiar to home care staff prior to their making any home visits.
3. All home care staff attend safety management inservice programs annually.	3. Annual refresher programs help to update staff and ensure compliance with standards.
4. The primary nurse is responsible for educating the patient/caregiver on home safety and providing them with the appropriate educational material. The patient and caregivers are instructed on safety measures specific to their individual needs.	4. Reviewing age-specific safety factors with all patients and caregivers helps to prevent unnecessary incidents.
5. The primary nurse assesses pertinent safety factors and documents the assessment and any instruction given, on the patient's record.	5. Documentation records the information covered with the patient in case any incident should occur in the future.
6. If any safety hazard, accident, incident, or injury occurs, the home care staff involved document the problem using the incident reporting mechanism.	6. All incidents must be reported to comply with agency and legal requirements.

7. Any incidents involving equipment malfunction, injury, or death associated with equipment are to be reported to the DME vendor and/or manufacturer immediately.

7. Malfunctioning of equipment is the responsibility of the equipment company, not the home care program.

Origin Date: _____
Revised Date: _____
Approved Date: _____
Originator: _____
Distribution: _____

1:61
SELECTION, ORIENTATION, AND EVALUATION OF PERSONNEL

PURPOSE:

To establish policies in conjunction with the personnel department regarding the selection, orientation and evaluation of personnel

RESPONSIBLE PERSONNEL:

Administrative and supervisory staff, personnel department

OBJECTIVES:

- To provide guidance to supervisory staff on the selection, orientation, and evaluation of personnel
- To ensure consistency with hospital personnel policies

POLICY:

- Staff performance is evaluated against job descriptions. The job description forms the basis for the criteria-based performance appraisal system. Staff are evaluated after the introductory period and annually. Home health aides are evaluated and competency tested annually.
- The home care department of Abington Memorial Hospital is required to comply with all hospital personnel policies and procedures. The administrative staff work closely with the personnel department in the selection and hiring of new employees. The home care department conducts an extensive departmental orientation. Staff are also required to attend a short hospital orientation.

PROCEDURE:

Action

Rationale

Selection of Employees

1. Personnel department forwards an employment application, which includes job history, and an interview assessment form

1. To maintain consistency with hospital procedure.

to the department. In addition, the home care department will accept applicants directly for select positions. (RN and home health aide only).
2. The department interviewer schedules and conducts the interview and completes the interview assessment form.
3. The applications and interview assessment forms of candidates who are not acceptable are returned to the personnel department.
4. The department interviewer discusses final candidate with personnel department.
5. The personnel department schedules an interview and formally offers the candidate the position.
6. The personnel department is responsible for obtaining two references and completing necessary paperwork.

2. Enables the interviewer to verify education, experience, training, and certification.
3. Personnel notifies candidates who are not accepted for the position.
4. Candidate's qualifications are discussed to ascertain salary.
5. Meets hospital policy.
6. The personnel department maintains employee personnel files. In addition, the home care department may choose to obtain references directly. Home care references are documented, sent to personnel department, and placed in home care department files.

Orientation of Personnel

1. Staff are required to attend specific components of hospital orientation.
2. All staff and contractors complete an orientation program specific to their position and responsibilities as well as agency's operation.

1. Ensures consistency in meeting hospital Joint Commission requirements.
2. An extensive orientation for newly appointed members of the staff/contractors will facilitate adjustments to the agency environment and job responsibilities.

Evaluation of Personnel

1. Criteria-based job descriptions and performance appraisals are developed for all personnel.
2. Management staff are evaluated based on the managerial performance appraisal. The development of individual goals and objectives relates to specific criteria within the job description.
3. Hourly employees are evaluated at the completion of the probationary period and annually thereafter.
    - RN staff: Clinical staff are evaluated annually. Skills and competence of staff are evaluated annually during supervised home visits. Staff are en-

1. Job descriptions form the basis by which staff are evaluated.
2. Managerial performance appraisals correlate with the hospital's wage/salary program. Annual increases are based 100 percent on performance.
3. Meets hospital policy.

- The in-home competency evaluation tool is an integral part of the performance appraisal process. Staff are evaluated and competency tested on

couraged to complete a self-evaluation.
- Home health aides: Home health aides are competency tested annually during supervised home visits and evaluated annually.

4. Social work (salaried) employees are evaluated at the probationary period and annually during the hospital's wage and salary program. Skills and competence of staff are evaluated annually during supervised home visits.

5. Contract workers (therapists) are evaluated annually prior to the renewal of the contract. Skills and competency are evaluated during supervised home visits.

6. Salaried employees are evaluated at the probationary period annually during the hospital's wage and salary program. Competency testing is completed as per Policy 1:13.

7. Supervisors are encouraged to use critical incident reports to facilitate the annual performance appraisal process.

job and/or age-specific criteria. (See Policy 1:13.)

4. The in-home competency evaluation tool is an integral part of the performance appraisal process. Staff are evaluated and competency tested on job and/or age-specific criteria. (See Policy 1:13.)

5. The in-home competency evaluation tool is an integral part of the performance appraisal process. Staff are evaluated and competency tested on job and/or age-specific criteria. (See Policy 1:13.)

6. Salaried employee's performance appraisal correlates with the wage and salary program. Annual increases are based 100 percent on performance.

7. Provides a tool to address with staff problems or deficiencies from a variety of sources, such as record review, patient complains, and QAI activities.

Origin Date: _____
Revised Date: _____
Approved Date: _____
Originator: _____
Distribution: _____

1:62
SOCIAL WORK SERVICES

PURPOSE:

To provide a description of the scope of practice of social work services in the home care/hospice program

RESPONSIBLE PERSONNEL:

Director of professional services, hospice coordinator, social workers

OBJECTIVES:

- To assess the patient's psychosocial and emotional needs
- To offer direct social services to individuals and families referred by agency professional staff to aid in the resolution of psychosocial difficulties that may interfere with the achievement of optimal benefits from current health care services
- To develop and maintain patient and/or staff liaison with other social and health resources and assist in their utilization as indicated

- To assist with integration of social services within the agency and development of an agency-wide consultation program
- To contribute to agency staff education through planned inservice programs and individual social guidance, instruction, and counseling
- To participate in development of the plan of care, discharge plan, audit evaluation, and utilization review
- To delineate qualifications of the social worker responsible for the provision of care (refer to job description)

POLICY:

- Social casework is a patient care service that enhances the agency services by providing direct patient/family assistance in coping with difficult psychosocial situations that may pose a threat to health status, makes appropriate social agency referrals, offers overall social service program support, and, subsequently, allows the nurse or other health personnel greater opportunity for more comprehensive care.
- Direct social work services will be provided to patients with supportive instruction and counseling to family, involved friends, and other agency personnel involved in the patient's care when the following criteria exist:
  - Patient must be currently admitted to the agency service.
  - The physician's written order must be obtained for social service.
  - Service priority will be offered where social problems hinder solution of an acute, serious health problem, existing psychosocial problems accompanied by the health problem present potential for solution through the agency's social services or by its referral to another agency, social service intervention will enhance the patient/family ability to use other available social services, and no other community/institutional social services are involved.
  - Services will be terminated in the following circumstances:
    (1) Mutual goals are not met within a reasonable time.
    (2) Patient/family fail in carrying out prescribed regimen.
    (3) Basic facilities conducive to a healthy environment become inadequate.
    (4) Patient/family or physician request termination of service if no longer required.
    (5) A change in patient's physical condition requires care or services not provided by the home health agency and referral is made to the proper agency for further care.
    (6) Physician is no longer directing care and medical treatment is refused.
    (7) Physician's orders are not renewed in accordance with established policy.
    (8) Physician and nurse/therapist mutually agree that goals have been met.
    (9) Patient's discharge reason is transfer to a hospital, skilled nursing facility, or another community agency.
    (10) Patient's residence is changed to a geographic area not served by the agency.
    (11) Patient/family refuse service and physician is notified.
    (12) Patient expires.

PROCEDURE:

Action	Rationale
Social work services are provided by qualified social workers in accordance with the plan of treatment signed by the physician. Social workers carry out the following functions.	These measures constitute the scope of social work services in a home care setting and comply with Medicare Conditions of Participation.

Direct Service

1. Complete social service assessment.
2. Provide direct social work services to patients.
3. Make referrals to other community services as indicated by the patient's needs.
4. Perform supportive instruction and counseling to family members and/or involved friends.

Consultation Service

1. Provide office consultation to the nurse or other agency personnel and/or make field visits to coordinate social work services.

Documentation

1. Complete the social service assessment.
2. Reassess the patient's and family's status on each visit, documenting in the progress note.
3. Develop the written plan within five days of social work services.
4. Revise the plan on an as-needed basis and incorporate revisions in the clinical note.
5. Review the plan with any other involved disciplines and reviews the plan of care with the physician every 62 days, or according to insurance guidelines.
6. Obtain verbal orders as indicated by the patient's changing status. (Refer to Policy 1:43, Medical Services.)
7. Keep complete and accurate clinical notes on all patients receiving therapy.
8. Record all field consultations and evaluations.
9. Provide all pertinent communication regarding the patient's care, progress, and status to the appropriate persons.
10. Conference with nurses and other disciplines involved in the patient's care.

Origin Date: _____
Revised Date: _____
Approved Date: _____
Originator: _____
Distribution: _____

1:63
SPEECH PATHOLOGY SERVICES

PURPOSE:

To provide a description of the scope of practice of the speech pathology services in the home care/hospice program (in accordance with the Pennsylvania Standards of Practice)

RESPONSIBLE PERSONNEL:

Director of professional services, therapy supervisor, hospice coordinator, speech pathologists

OBJECTIVES:

- To provide palliative speech therapy services
- To promote community understanding of speech therapy services
- To assist in the coordination of activities with AMHHC personnel and other community agencies in bringing about such physical, psychological, sound economic and vocational adjustments as may be indicated in the best interest of the patient
- To assist the patient in adjustment to the disability by:
  - assisting the patient in planning modifications to his or her surroundings and in achieving maximum physical independence
  - providing assistance to the family in the adjustment to the disability

POLICY:

- Speech pathology is a patient care service providing comprehensive speech, language, dysphagia, and hearing rehabilitation. Qualified therapists work as members of the home care/hospice team in a community setting and provide service to patients based on the referral and written prescription of a physician. The professional practice of speech pathology is directed toward diagnosis and treatment of speech, language, dysphagia, and hearing disorders.
- A clinical fellow who has met the educational requirements for certificate of clinical competency in speech pathology and is currently complying with experience requirements for completion of the clinical fellowship year shall be under the supervision of a therapist.

PROCEDURE:

Action	Rationale
Speech pathology services are provided by qualified speech pathologists in accordance with the plan of treatment prescribed by a physician. This plan is based on the speech pathologist's assessment of the patient's level of functioning. Speech pathologists carry out the following functions.	These measures constitute the scope of speech therapy practicum in a home care setting and complies with Medicare Conditions of Participation.

Direct Service

1. Evaluate patients with a wide range of diagnoses, in accordance with the plan of treatment prescribed by a physician, using established clinical measurement procedures.
2. Formulate an assessment of patient's rehabilitation potential and treatment goals, and implement plan of therapy based on evaluation findings.
3. Provide written instructions to the patient, identifying activities to be carried out between visits.
4. Teach selected procedures to a responsible member of the family.
5. Assess total patient and family needs and, when necessary, make referrals to available community resources to meet those needs.

Consultation Service

1. Provide office consultation to the nurse and hospice IDG when necessary, and make joint field visits to coordinate speech pathology services for newly admitted patients or for patients who have a previously established plan of care from nursing or from the speech language pathologist.

Documentation

1. Complete an assessment and plan of care within five days.
2. Develop the written plan of care for speech language pathology services and obtain a signed plan of treatment from the physician.
3. Document written evaluations and review the plan of treatment with the physician every 62 days or according to hospice benefit periods.
4. Reassess the patient's status and progress on each visit and document in the clini-

cal note. Complete a new evaluation and plan of care after each hospitalization.
5. Obtain verbal orders as indicated by the patient's changing status and get follow-up signature from the physician. (Refer to Policy 1:43, Medical Services.)
6. Revise the plan as needed. Incorporate revisions in the clinical note.
7. Keep complete and accurate clinical notes on all patients receiving therapy.
8. Record all interdisciplinary consultation and family teaching.
9. Provide all pertinent communication regarding the patient's care, progress, and status to the appropriate persons.
10. Confer with nurses and hospice IDG.
11. Supervise clinical fellows and cosign all written notations in the medical record.

Origin Date: _____
Revised Date: _____
Approved Date: _____
Originator: _____
Distribution: _____

1:64
STAFF DEVELOPMENT

PURPOSE:

To ensure that there is growth, stimulation, motivation, and continued competence of all employees and contractors

RESPONSIBLE PERSONNEL:

Governing body, executive director, director of professional services, quality assessment and improvement supervisor, all staff

OBJECTIVES:
- To establish a working environment that is conducive to continued learning
- To inspire acceptance of individual responsibility for learning
- To introduce new knowledge and techniques to meet current standards, needs, and trends
- To provide orientation for all staff and contractors
- To provide inservice education programs for all levels of staff throughout the year
- To encourage individual employees/contractors to pursue continuing education courses
- To prepare a one-year calendar of tentative programs to be presented each year
- To include staff on a committee that plans educational experiences
- To provide resources to meet the need for knowledge-based information and literature

POLICY:

- Staff development is an essential component of a home health agency's quality assessment and improvement program. All staff/contractors will complete an orientation program and will document participation in inservice and continuing education programs during each fiscal year. Administration and staff share responsibility to support and promote learning experiences to ensure current knowledge and practice.
- The department maintains a library of journals, publications and audiovisual aids. All staff have access to information contained in the library, including patient education material. The administrative staff keep abreast of current trends and regulatory and legislative changes through review of national trade organization publications and journals and attendance at conferences and seminars.

PROCEDURE:

Action	Rationale
1. The governing body and administration will provide a framework, staff, and funds to facilitate an ongoing program.	1. Structural components must be in place and communicated to staff.
2. One individual is assigned the responsibility to coordinate the program.	2. One individual can schedule multiple activities on a master calendar and oversee the total program.
3. A staff development budget is included in agency budget and account for disbursements.	3. Funds must be authorized to carry out the activities.
4. A library is maintained within the agency.	4. Current reference books and professional journals need to be available in the agency.
5. All staff and contractors complete an orientation program specific to their position and responsibilities, as well as agency's operations.	5. An extensive orientation for newly appointed members of the staff/contractors will facilitate adjustment to the agency environment and job responsibilities.
6. Based on the needs of the staff, the organization, and federal accreditation and certification standards, inservice educational programs are scheduled on a regular basis. Topics address new or revised procedures and new product education are chosen to maintain competence. (See Policy 1:13, Competency Evaluation Program.)	6. The administrative and supervisory staff collect and analyze data to determine staff educational/competency needs. Such things as new program development, performance improvement, and performance evaluation problems are considered. The staff education committee meets regularly to address needs.
7. Attendees complete an evaluation form at the end of each session.	7. The evaluations provide objective analysis of programs.
8. Paid attendance at continuing programs is made available within the constraints of time and dollars.	8. Continuing education is a joint responsibility. Individuals must assume some responsibility for their educational experiences.

9. Staff and contractors complete an educational program record on an annual basis for personnel file.	9. Documentation provides evidence of educational activities.
10. Home health aides receive 12 hours of inservice training per calendar year. The inservice training may be provided while the aide is furnishing care to patients.	10. This training ensures compliance with Medicare Conditions of Participation.

Origin Date: _____
Revised Date: _____
Approved Date: _____
Originator: _____
Distribution: _____

1:65
SUPPORT GROUP

- A support group is available for the hospice team members to address issues such as staff stress, grieving, and clinical needs. The group is open to all professional team members and meets at the discretion of the hospice coordinator, or at least quarterly. The hospice IDG may initiate a request for additional support services. If the need arises, administration will consider the support group's request for additional external stress management and/or bereavement resources.
- Emphasis will be placed on the use of the support group as a constructive means to reduce stress associated with hospice patient care and to promote research in the area of stress management and patient care.
- In addition to the hospice support group, the AMH employee assistance program is available to provide individual counseling as needed.

Origin Date: _____
Revised Date: _____
Approved Date: _____
Originator: _____
Distribution: _____

1:66
TRANSFER TO OTHER SETTINGS

POLICY:
- If, on the basis of IDG evaluation and in consultation with the patient's family, the patient requires transfer to an acute or extended care facility, every effort will be made to ensure a smooth transition.
- To facilitate continuity of care for the hospice patient, the hospice program will provide a brief summary of home care to inpatient facilities.

- This summary will include a description of services provided, specific medications, and psychosocial or other problems requiring intervention and follow-up.

Origin Date: _____
Revised Date: _____
Approved Date: _____
Originator: _____
Distribution: _____

1:67
TWENTY-FOUR-HOUR SERVICE

PURPOSE:

To establish protocols for providing 24-hour service availability

RESPONSIBLE PERSONNEL:

Executive director, director of professional services, clinical supervisors, professional nursing staff

OBJECTIVES:

- To inform patients of availability of service 24 hours a day, dependent on need
- To establish criteria for the processing of calls outside regular office hours
- To establish measures to enhance staff safety when making visits after office hours
- To establish nurse coverage for all hours while creating optimum flexibility in scheduling

POLICY:

Service is available 24 hours a day, seven days a week. The following guidelines are observed:
- Patients are informed that 24-hour answering service is available and assured that someone will respond to their call.
- A nurse responds to all calls referred by the answering service and makes visits to patients, if indicated. Visits are made at the nurse's discretion in consultation with a hospice coordinator or clinical supervisor.
- Visits are made only to patients known to the service or who are newly referred by a physician.
- Visits are not made as a substitute for medical evaluation or treatment.
- Visits are not normally made for resolution of bowel problems. However, visits will be made for management of acute symptoms such as pain, severe nausea and vomiting, acute anxiety, and so forth.
- Visits are not normally made for routine replacement of leaking Foley catheters. Regarding diagnosis of urinary retention: Visits will be based on the time of the call and nurse's telephone assessment of patient's discomfort rather than just the diagnosis. Visits may be postponed until the beginning of the next day depending on the nurse's assessment.
- Care will be given in accordance with the established interdisciplinary group plan of care or after consultation with a physician.

- Preplanned visits after office hours are made as scheduled.
- For hospice benefit patients, nursing services, physician services, and drugs and biologicals are routinely available on a 24-hour basis. Other covered services, such as medical, social worker, chaplain, medical supplies, inpatient care, continuous care, and so forth, are available on a 24-hour basis to the extent necessary to meet the needs of individuals for care that is reasonable and necessary for the palliation and management of terminal illness and related conditions.

PROCEDURE:

Action	Rationale
1. All patients are notified of the 24-hour answering service when admitted.	1. This assures patients that a nurse is always available to respond to their needs.
2. The answering service refers all requests for service to the nurse on call.	2. The nurse determines if a visit is needed.
3. The nurse makes a decision as to necessity for a visit, consulting with a hospice coordinator or clinical supervisor as indicated.	3. Every attempt is made to provide adequate intervention based on the patient's stated needs.
4. For unscheduled visits, the nurse contacts the hospice coordinator or clinical supervisor before leaving home and upon returning home, as indicated.	4. These measures help to ensure the safety of the nurse making visits outside regular office hours.
5. The nurse wears a name badge/identification and adheres to dress code to make all visits.	5. These measures help to ensure the safety of the nurse making visits outside regular office hours.
6. If the nurse or supervisor has any concern about the safety of the nurse making the visit, security is contacted to escort the nurse.	6. These measures help to ensure the safety of the nurse making visits outside regular office hours.
7. The nurses are scheduled to work on evenings, nights, and weekends on a rotating basis. The nurse scheduled may make arrangements for another nurse to substitute for him or her.	7. This provides for nurse coverage for all hours while creating flexibility for nurses to meet personal needs.
8. Time sheets are completed for all time worked and visits made, including the start and stop time of visit, reason, patient's name, nurse who makes visit, and indication of whether visit is scheduled or unscheduled.	8. Time sheets provide data for analysis of services rendered outside of regular office hours and generate payroll data.

Origin Date: _____
Revised Date: _____
Approved Date: _____
Originator: _____
Distribution: _____

1:68
UTILIZATION REVIEW

PURPOSE:

To evaluate the appropriateness of client admissions and discharges, appropriate utilization of levels and types of personnel, and over- and underutilization of services

PROCEDURES:

1. The quality assessment/performance improvement committee will review randomly selected clinical records for over- and underutilization of services on a quarterly basis. At least 10 percent of hospice patients will be reviewed as part of the quarterly record review and utilization review. All hospice benefit patients will be reviewed for utilization, per the quality assessment/performance improvement record review process.
2. The quality assessment/performance improvement committee reviews clinical records on a quarterly basis per quarterly record review policy and procedure. The utilization review report is completed on cases in which there are questions of either under- or overutilization. Reports are presented to the quality assessment/performance improvement supervisor for further investigation.
3. Based on the above reviews, a summary report is presented to the professional advisory committee that discusses appropriate utilization of all clinical services.

Origin Date: _____
Revised Date: _____
Approved Date: _____
Originator: _____
Distribution: _____

1:69
VERIFICATION OF PHYSICIAN'S LICENSE

PURPOSE:

To establish procedure to verify and document physician's license in order to meet Joint Commission on Accreditation for Healthcare Organizations accreditation standards

RESPONSIBLE PERSONNEL:

Executive director, director of professional services, clerical staff

OBJECTIVES:

To ensure that medical care is prescribed by a licensed physician

POLICY:

Physicians who refer patients to the organization and from whom orders are accepted must have their licenses verified, and documentation of the verification must be on file.

PROCEDURE:

Action	Rationale
1. The clerical staff maintain on file a list of physicians' names and license numbers. This list is updated periodically as new physicians make referrals for service.	1. These measures ensure that the licenses of all referring physicians are valid and provide the necessary documentation to meet Joint Commission accreditation standards.
2. Upon admission of a patient, the clerical staff check the list to verify that the referring physician is licensed.	2. This measure ensures that the licenses of all referring physicians are valid and provide the necessary documentation to meet Joint Commission accreditation standards.
3. If the referring physician's name does not appear on the list, the clerical staff verify the license number by telephoning the appropriate county or state medical society, or the state board of medical examiners.	3. This measure ensures that the licenses of all referring physicians are valid and provide the necessary documentation to meet Joint Commission accreditation standards.

Origin Date: _____
Revised Date: _____
Approved Date: _____
Originator: _____
Distribution: _____

1:70
VIOLENCE/NEGLECT/ABUSE

PURPOSE:

To facilitate referral for patients identified to be at risk for injury or neglect

RESPONSIBLE PERSONNEL:

All clinical and supervisory personnel, including nurses, physical therapists, occupational therapists, speech therapists, social workers, chaplains, dietitians and home health aides

POLICY:

- The home care department acknowledges the responsibility of all clinical personnel to identify abuse and/or serious neglect in the home and to take necessary available steps to protect the safety of patients and others.
- The clinical supervisor is to be informed of the suspected abuse and/or neglect as soon as possible. In addition, the medical social worker should be consulted for further support, clinical involvement, and evaluation.

- The primary goal of this policy is to provide for the safety of patients and others by assisting the patient in connecting with service organizations voluntarily. Should the patient refuse voluntary referral and should law allow, mandatory referral will be pursued through social service organizations dealing with issues of abuse and neglect. Abuse situations likely to be identified include adult or pediatric patients at risk of violence, neglect, or financial exploitation at the hands of others.

PROCEDURE:

Action	Rationale
1. Patients shall be assessed for risk of abuse or neglect. The following criteria should be considered when assessing for abuse or neglect. *Adult* - Injuries to the trunk of the body that indicate they could be intentional as compared to a distally located injury indicating a possible accident - Any injury with a patterned appearance to it such as marks from a belt or ring - Bruised skin from a grasp - Any patient who reports an abusive accident - Lack of appropriate medication - Lack of food supply - Substandard housing - Lack of adequate caregiver for dependent patient *Child* - Parents who were abused themselves - Burns caused from scalding - An imprint from a hot object on the back, buttocks, or back of the hands - Fracture that does not correlate with the child's gross motor ability - Femoral fractures in children younger than two years - Rib fractures in infants and children	1. Complete assessment of psychosocial issues forms the basis for holistic care and the provision of safety to all patients. The domestic violence computer help screen will assist staff in formulating appropriate questioning to facilitate the assessment.
2. All patients found to be at serious risk for injury/neglect to self or others shall be urged to seek immediate voluntary referral to appropriate community agencies.	2. Voluntary action on the part of patients to protect themselves or others is the preferred means for providing safe, appropriate care.

3. All patients found to be at serious risk of injury/neglect to self or others and who refuse to seek voluntary assessment/treatment shall be advised that action can or will be taken to initiate contact with appropriate community agencies as state law allows.

4. All patient situations of serious injury/neglect shall be discussed as soon as possible with the clinical supervisor, medical social worker, and the patient's physician for further assistance and support. The social worker shall be responsible for assessing and initiating referrals as situations come to light during usual business hours. After usual business hours, the staff person shall seek guidance from the on-call nursing supervisor.

5. All clinical staff entering a home shall be apprised of the risk of injury to the patient or themselves when such risk is known, and every effort shall be made to uphold staff safety, including use of the escort service as needed.

6. Requests for assistance in dealing with issues of voluntary referral will be directed to the appropriate community agencies by the social worker.

3. When voluntary action by the patient is refused, involuntary action to protect the patient or others must be instituted in accordance with state law for population age groups protected by law.

4. All available resources shall be used to provide timely attention to the patient/family and support for staff involved in a stressful situation. The social worker's skills and assessment, counseling, and referral will benefit patients in a time of trauma.

5. Staff safety is of paramount importance. Communication will ensure that these goals are attained.

6. Current legislation does not allow intervention without patient consent for competent adults. Staff will encourage patients to allow referral to protect their own safety and that of others. Efforts will be made to use existing legal resources in doing so. If a question of patient competence arises, staff will contact the appropriate agency for direction, and will refer to the policy on psychiatric emergencies.

Origin Date: _____
Revised Date: _____
Approved Date: _____
Originator: _____
Distribution: _____

1:71
VOLUNTEER RECRUITMENT AND RETENTION

POLICY:

- Volunteer recruitment is ongoing throughout the year. The director of volunteers records recruitment activities and relays the documentation to the executive director.
- Efforts toward retention of volunteers are made through monthly support meetings, incorporating educational programs, resource speakers, and individual counseling.

Origin Date: _____
Revised Date: _____
Approved Date: _____
Originator: _____
Distribution: _____

1:72
VOLUNTEER SERVICES

PURPOSE:

To provide volunteer health and related services to the professional team members and patients in the agency's various areas of service

RESPONSIBLE PERSONNEL:

Executive director, volunteer director, assistant coordinator and volunteers

OBJECTIVES:

- To provide the health team with direct or indirect supplemental assistance
- To plan and implement a quality program
- To recruit, select, coordinate, and supervise volunteers
- To evaluate and recommend methods to improve the volunteer program

POLICY:

The agency is committed to the development and the implementation of a quality volunteer program. It is a multifaceted program that encompasses an ongoing evaluation by patients, volunteers, and administrators.

PROCEDURE:

Action	Rationale
1. Recruit volunteers through advertisement, public speaking engagements, brochures, and networking in other organizations.	1. An adequate supply of quality volunteers must be maintained.
2. Select volunteers by interview and screening qualifications without regard for age, sex, or race.	2. In selection, sincerity of purpose and individual ability should take precedence.

3. Plan and implement an on-site formal orientation course and monthly inservices presented by volunteer director and/or qualified professionals.
4. Assign volunteers to provide direct or indirect health services with consideration of individual preferences and ability.
5. Supervise and teach volunteers in basic procedures, and offer guidance in assuming responsibilities of assigned areas or in providing direct patient services.
6. Instruct volunteers in documentation of services rendered and time contributed, and ensure that documentation is obtained.
7. Evaluate periodically the performance of the volunteers and program by telephone calls, questionnaires, or visits to patients' homes.
8. Provide for annual recognition of volunteer services.
9. Terminate services of volunteer if, in the department's opinion, this action is in everyone's best interest.

3. An ongoing teaching program should be provided for the volunteers, encompassing philosophy, methodology, and skills required.
4. The department should supply health services and patients with appropriate volunteers.
5. Quality performance is needed from the volunteers in all areas.
6. Adequate patient records must be maintained. The volunteer is an important member of the care team. Information needs to be communicated to other team members. Volunteer time is credited to the volunteer and the program.
7. The department needs to determine that goals are being met. Evaluation also provides feedback.
8. Positive feedback should be provided to all individuals who donate their time for the department and its patients.
9. Multiple absences or failure to comply with general department rules and volunteer regulations are not conducive to continued volunteer services.

Origin Date: _____
Revised Date: _____
Approved Date: _____
Originator: _____
Distribution: _____

1:73
WITHDRAWAL OF LIFE-SUSTAINING CARE

PURPOSE:

To establish a policy and procedure concerning the withdrawal of life-sustaining care

RESPONSIBLE PERSONNEL:

Visiting staff and supervisory staff, patient's attending physician

OBJECTIVES:

To establish a consistent policy to address the withdrawal of life-sustaining care

POLICY:

- It is the policy of Abington Memorial Hospital to honor a patient's advance directive regarding DNR (do not resuscitate) orders and/or the withdrawal of life-sustaining treatment. A physician's order is required to implement an advance directive. Staff are required to comply with policies for DNR orders with or without an advance directive.
- Information regarding hospice policies is contained in the Patient Bill of Rights and the Advance Directive Brochure.

PROCEDURE:

Action

1. Refer to Do Not Resuscitate Policy (1:20) and Advance Directives Policy (1:06).

Rationale

1. The advance directive is the mechanism by which patients express their wishes regarding the withdrawal of life-sustaining care. State law requires a physician's order to implement.

Origin Date: _____
Revised Date: _____
Approved Date: _____
Originator: _____
Distribution: _____

PART II

Forms

Table of Contents

Form	Form Number	COP
Acute Inpatient Care	1	418.56(e)
Annual Administrative Review	2	418.52
Assessment of Bereavement Risk	3	418.88(a)
Bereavement Assessment	4	418.88(a)
Bereavement Follow-Up	5	418.88(a)
Change of Designated Hospice	6	418.30
Consent for Release of Information	7	418.74
Critical Incident Report	8	418.66
Departmental Incident Report Tracking Form	9	418.66
Election of Hospice Medicare Benefit—Informed Consent	10	418.21, 418.62
General Transfer Form	11	418.56
Hospice Charts—Filing Sequence	12	418.74
Hospice Contractor Orientation Program	13	418.56, 418.64
Hospice Discharge Checklist: Inpatient	14	418.74
Hospice Discharge Checklist: Routine and Inpatient Records	15	418.74
Hospice Discharge Checklist: Routine Services	16	418.74
Hospice Home Visit Consent Form	17	418.62
Hospice Medicare Benefit Revocation	18	418.28
Hospice Volunteer Bereavement Training Syllabus	19	418.70, 418.88
Interdisciplinary Care Plan	20	418.58
MSW Competency—In-Home Evaluation	21	418.56, 418.64
Nursing Competency—In-Home Evaluation	22	418.56, 418.64
Orientation Program	23	418.64
Pain Assessment	24	418.82
Patient Consent for Care	25	418.62
Physician Certification/Recertification of Terminal Illness	26	418.22

Plan of Care for Inpatient Respite	27	418.56(e)
Quality Assurance Quarterly Record Review Nursing (Hospice)	28	418.66
Resource List—Religious Groups	29	418.70(f), 418.88
Resource List—Suggested Readings on Death, Dying, Bereavement	30	418.88
Spiritual/Religious Assessment	31	418.70(f), 418.88(c)
Therapy Competency In-Home Evaluation	32	418.56
Volunteer Assessment and Plan: Inpatient Unit	33	418.70
Volunteer Training Program Syllabus	34	418.70

FORM 1

ACUTE INPATIENT CARE

Patient Name: _____ Admission Date: _____

Diagnosis: _____ Physician: _____

Reason for Transfer: _____

Description of Patient's General Condition: _____

_____

_____

Current Medications: _____

_____

_____

Recommended Orders for Services and Treatments:

Diet: _____ Activity: _____ Oxygen: _____

Skin care/wound treatment: _____

Other: _____

_____

PHYSICIAN CERTIFICATION: I/We certify/recertify that the above patient is terminally ill with a life expectancy of six months or less.

DO NOT RESUSCITATE: In the event of cardiac or respiratory arrest, CPR (Cardiopulmonary resuscitation) measures will not be initiated.

Special Considerations: _____

Hospice Visit Schedule: _____

Does the patient have an advance directive? _____

If no, was information on obtaining one provided? _____

Signature: _____ Date: _____

Hospice Medical Director: _____

Hospice Coordinator: _____

COP 418.56(e)

FORM 2

ANNUAL ADMINISTRATIVE REVIEW

The annual administrative review of the Abington Memorial Hospital's Home Care Department Policy and Procedure Manual for the hospice program was completed. New policies have been included; existing policies have been updated. Policies and procedures have also been reviewed and approved by the interdisciplinary team. These changes are shared with the professional advisory committee as well as with the staff. The minutes of the interdisciplinary group (IDG) committee reflect the actions taken at these meetings.

_____
Executive Director

_____
Hospice Coordinator

_____
Executive Vice President
Abington Memorial Hospital

_____
Date

COP 418.52

FORM 3

ASSESSMENT OF BEREAVEMENT RISK

1. What was the length of time in the relationship between the bereaved and the deceased?
    (1) 0–10 years (2) 11–20 years (3) 21 or more years
2. Do you perceive that a dysfunctional relationship existed between the bereaved and the deceased?
    (1) Not obvious (2) Possibly (3) Apparent
3. Is the bereaved expressing despair/depression or thoughts of suicide?
    (1) Never (2) Occasionally (3) Often
4. How emotionally well supported is the bereaved (family, friends, religion)?
    (1) Well supported (2) Somewhat supported (3) Unsupported
5. How easily can the bereaved discuss his or her feelings with support staff, family, or friends?
    (1) Easily (2) Needs encouragement (3) Has difficulty
6. Has the bereaved experienced other recent losses within the past two years?
    (1) 0 persons (2) 1 person (3) 2 or more persons
7. Is the bereaved using drugs or alcohol?
    (1) Never (2) Same as before (3) More frequently than before
8. Does the bereaved have any current medical problems?
    (1) None (2) Several (3) Numerous
9. Has the bereaved's physical status been adversely affected by the loss, for example, appetite, weight loss or gain, sleeping habits?
    (1) Not affected (2) Somewhat affected (3) Noticeably affected
10. Will the bereaved's lifestyle be adversely affected by the loss, for example, financial, housing, employment?
    (1) Not affected (2) Somewhat affected (3) Substantially affected

SCORING

Risk Factors: Low: 10–15
               Medium: 16–25
               High: 26–30

Low Risk: Normal grief and reconciliation. Follow regular bereavement plan.
Medium Risk: May need additional support. Monitor.
High Risk: Requires additional support. Monitor closely for possible referral and intervention.

Sources: Compiled from Lehigh Hospice Risk Assessment Tool and other materials.

COP 418.88(a)

FORM 4

BEREAVEMENT ASSESSMENT

Name of Deceased: _____   Date of Death: _____
Birth Date: _____   Medical Record No.: _____
Hospice Adm. Date: _____   Bereaved's Phone No.: _____

_____

1. Name of Bereaved _____ 2. Age _____ 3. Sex _____
4. Address _____
_____
5. Relationship to Patient: _____ 6. Length of Relationship: _____
_____
7. How long was illness? _____
8. Place of death: Hospice _____ Home _____ Nursing Home _____ Other _____
   Circumstances of death: Expected _____ Sudden _____ Other _____
9. Support system: Family _____ Friends _____ Religion/church _____
10. Physical status.
    a. Appetite: _____ b. Weight loss/gain _____
    c. Change in sleeping habits? Yes _____ No _____ Describe _____
    d. How is the bereaved's general health? _____
11. Is the bereaved interested in receiving bereavement materials? Yes _____ No: _____
12. Others needing bereavement support:
    Name: _____
    Address: _____ Phone No. _____
13. Comments or concerns:
    _____
    _____

14. Bereavement Protocol: For Office Use Only
    _____ Sent sympathy card
    _____ Sent bereavement materials
    _____ Scheduled regular bereavement phone call support
    _____ Scheduled individual support for high-risk client
    _____ Bereavement support declined by bereaved
    _____ Invited to support group
    _____ Invited to memorial service

Date assessment completed: _____ Call length of time: _____

Signature of Assessor: _____ Volunteer No.: _____

COP 418.88(a)

FORM 5

BEREAVEMENT FOLLOW-UP

Name of Deceased: _____ Date of Death: _____
Birth Date: _____ Medical Record No.: _____
Hospice Adm. Date: _____ Bereaved's Phone No.: _____
Follow up in: Jan Feb Mar Apr May Jun Jul Aug Sep Oct Nov Dec
Additional calls as needed (give date): _____

1. Name of Bereaved _____ 2. Age _____ 3. Sex _____
4. Address _____
_____
5. Relationship to Patient: _____ 6. Length of Relationship: _____
7. Type of Contact: Visit_____ Phone Call _____ Letter _____
8. Physical status:
   a. Appetite: _____ b. Weight loss/gain _____
   c. Change in sleeping habits? Yes _____ No _____ Describe _____
   d. How is the bereaved's general health? _____
   e. Alcohol or drugs (change in habits)? _____
9. Is the bereaved interested in receiving bereavement materials? Yes _____ No _____
10. Emotional status:
   a. Guilt: Yes_____ No_____ b. Anger: Yes_____ No_____
   Comments: _____
_____
   c. Depression: Yes_____ No_____ d. Lonely/isolated: Yes_____ No_____
   e. Thoughts of suicide: Yes_____ No_____
   Comments: _____
_____

11. Continuity of Previous Lifestyle:
   a. Financial _____
   b. Housing _____
   c. Employment _____
12. Emotional support (family, friends, religion): _____
_____
13. Comments or concerns: _____
_____
_____
14. Referral or intervention indicated: Yes_____ No_____

Date assessment completed: _____ Call length of time: _____

Signature of Assessor: _____ Volunteer No.: _____

COP 418.88(a)

FORM 6

CHANGE OF DESIGNATED HOSPICE

Effective _____, I choose to designate a new hospice program from which I wish to
           (Date)

receive care.

1. On the above date I no longer wish to receive care from Abington Memorial Hospital Home Care Hospice. On this date, I plan to receive care from _____ Hospice.
2. It has been confirmed that I can be admitted to the _____ Hospice program on the above date.
3. I understand that this change will not reduce in any way the hospice Medicare benefits to which I am entitled.

_____   _____
Date   Signature of Patient or Legal Representative

_____   _____
Date   Witness Signature

COP 418.30

FORM 7

CONSENT FOR RELEASE OF INFORMATION

1. I authorize Abington Memorial Hospital Home Care Hospice Program to release information from, or copies of, my hospice medical record and/or to allow review by the following reimbursement sources:

   _____
   _____
   _____

2. I understand that the above release of information is required for the purpose of obtaining reimbursement for hospice care provided. I am authorizing release of all future medical record documentation relating to my hospice care to those sources named above. This authorization will not be valid once the above-named sources have received copies of and/or reviewed my medical record to verify any claim received or payment made to Abington Memorial Hospital Home Care Hospice Program.
3. I understand that the reimbursement sources listed cannot release to anyone else any information received unless I specifically authorize such a release.
4. In the event I am rehospitalized at Abington Memorial Hospital, I authorize the release of my hospital record for any documentation the hospice requires (per Medicare regulation) to the Abington Memorial Hospital Home Care Hospice Program.

_____   _____
Date   Signature of Patient or Legal Representative

_____   _____
Date   Witness Signature

COP 418.74

FORM 8

CRITICAL INCIDENT REPORT

NAME _____ DATE _____ UNIT _____

1. Describe the occurrence, including date, time, location, and outcomes. State the facts and whether they were observed by you (the manager) or reported to you: _____
   _____
   _____
   _____
   _____
   _____

2. Describe the action taken by the supervisor: _____
   _____
   _____
   _____

3. Expectations for improvement/follow-up: _____
   _____
   _____
   _____

4. Employee comments: _____
   _____

I have read and understand the above.   Verbal Warning: Yes _____ No _____

Date _____ Employee Signature _____

Date _____ Supervisor Signature _____

COP 418.66

FORM 9

DEPARTMENTAL INCIDENT REPORT TRACKING FORM

Patient Name: _____ Date of Occurrence: _____

Type of Occurrence:
_____ Infection secondary to care/treatment
_____ Staff infection (e.g., hepatitis, tuberuclosis, scabies, etc.)
_____ Workplace violence in the office or home
_____ Medication error and/or significant drug reactions
_____ Equipment malfunction:
      Name of equipment: _____
      Manufacturer: _____
      Model No.: _____
      Serial No.: _____
      Lot No.: _____
      DME Company: _____

Additional Pertinent Details on Occurrence: _____
_____
_____
_____

Contributing Factors/Cause of Occurrence: _____
_____
_____

Immediate Corrective Action: _____
_____
_____

Measures Taken To Prevent Recurrence of Event: _____
_____
_____

Opportunities for Improvement: **RISE** to the challenge. Check one or more boxes below.
_____ **R**ecurring event: Trend/pattern noted.
_____ **I**solated or single event: No trend noted.
_____ **S**entinel event: More intensive follow-up pending.
_____ **E**ducation/retraining needed.
     Specify: _____

Manager Supervisor: _____ Date: _____

Department Head: _____ Date: _____

COP 418.66

FORM 10

ELECTION OF HOSPICE MEDICARE BENEFIT—INFORMED CONSENT

Name: _____ Patient No.:_____

Address: _____
_____

I ACKNOWLEDGE/UNDERSTAND THE FOLLOWING:

I understand the nature of hospice care available through the hospice Medicare benefit and am aware that all treatment will be palliative rather than curative in nature. Treatment will be for management of symptoms and to provide for my terminal illness of_____ .

I understand that my care will be provided by a hospice team composed of a physician, nurse, social worker, pastoral counselor, volunteer, and other disciplines that may be necessary.

I waive the right to all other benefits under the Medicare program while I am receiving hospice benefits. Only Abington Memorial Hospital Home Care Hospice Program will be able to receive Medicare payment for care or services provided to me for my illness or any other condition *related* to my terminal illness.

Medicare will make payments for unlimited hospice days. However, the days are broken into three benefit periods to be used in this order: These periods are as follows:
    First Benefit Period—90 days
    Second Benefit Period—90 days
    Unlimited Benefit Period—Renewed every 60 days

I understand that I can use standard Medicare in the usual manner to pay the bill of
    1. My physician, if he or she is not an employee of this hospice
    2. Treatment of a condition *unreleated* to my terminal illness (see above)

I understand that I can revoke this benefit at any time and resume regular Medicare coverage. I know I will lose any hospice days remaining in the benefit period in which I revoke.

ACKNOWLEDGING/UNDERSTANDING THE ABOVE, I AUTHORIZE HOSPICE MEDICARE COVERAGE TO BEGIN ON _____ (Month/Day/Year).

_____   _____
Date of Signature   Signature or Legal Representative

    _____
    Relationship of Legal Representative to Beneficiary

_____   _____
Date of Signature   Witness Signature

COP 418.21, 418.62

FORM 11

GENERAL TRANSFER FORM

To: _____   Patient Name: _____
      (Facility/Contact Person)

_____   _____
      (Address)   (Address)

_____   _____
      (Telephone)   (Telephone)

    Patient _____ has been receiving skilled services from Abington Memorial Hospital Home Care Hospice.

    To ensure continuity of care, we are providing you with the following information. Please notify Abington Memorial Hospital Home Care Hospice if the patient should require our services in the future.

Thank you.

Reason for transfer/referral: _____
Mental, physical, and psychosocial status: _____
_____

V/S range: Pulse _____ Resp._____ Temp._____ BP_____
Services received: SN_____ PT_____ OT_____ ST_____ HHA_____ MSW_____ Hospice_____
Patient mental status: _____
Caregiver status and ability: _____
Patient has an advance directive_____   Patient does not have an advance directive_____
Summary of care, special treatments, limitations to care at home, progress toward goal achievement, instructions provided: _____
_____

Date _____ Signature _____

COP 418.56

FORM 12

HOSPICE CHARTS—FILING SEQUENCE

LEFT SIDE—FRONT TO BACK

1. Master File Input (MFI) Card (at discharge)
2. Verbal Orders
3. Interdisciplinary Care Plan (orders)
   A. IDG POC for continuous care nursing (if available)
   B. IDG POC for inpatient respite
   C. IDG POC for acute inpatient services
4. Physician Certification of Terminal Illness—Medicare, or Department of Public Welfare for Medical Assistance Benefit
5. Election of Hospice—Medicare Benefit, or Department of Public Welfare (Medical Assistance Benefit)
6. Hospice Program Patient Consent for Care (*all charts*)
7. Consent for release of information (*all charts*)
8. Master File Input Form (copy)
9. Assessment forms (MSW, PT, OT, ST)
10. Spiritual/Religious Assessment
11. Advance Directive (if available)
12. Home Health Aide POC and POC for Respite Shift (if available)
13. Volunteer Assessment and Plan
14. Referral for Services (if available)
15. Authorization and Release (copy from home care record)
16. Bill of Rights (copy from home care record)
17. Medicare Secondary Payer Questionnaire
18. Home Health Aide Activity Records
19. Miscellaneous—Lab reports, faxes, change in level of care

RIGHT SIDE—FRONT TO BACK

1. Patient Master Update I (PMUI) (following discharge)
2. Revocation of Hospice Care (Medicare or Medical Assistance, if available)
3. Change of Designated Hospice (Medicare or Medical Assistance, if available)
4. Discharge Summary
5. Progress Notes (newest on top)
   A. Yellow—Nursing
   B. Pink—Physical Therapy
   C. Gold—Occupational Therapy
   D. Blue—Speech Therapy
   E. Green—Social Service
   F. White—Chaplain
   G. Cream—Volunteers
6. Flow Sheets
7. Medication List (copy from home care chart)
8. Nutrition Assessment
9. Braden Pressure Ulcer Risk Assessment
10. Nursing Assessment (copy from home care chart)

COP 418.74

FORM 13

HOSPICE CONTRACTOR ORIENTATION PROGRAM

Name: _____ Date: _____
Position: _____

                                                                                       Date   Signature

I. Orientation to hospice structure
    A. Introduction to hospice program
        1. Philosophy
        2. Organizational structure
        3. Introduction to administrative, office, and clinical personnel and facilities
        4. Geographic area served
        5. Scope of services: total program and services provided
    B. Personnel policies: review and discussion
        1. Payment procedure
        2. Schedule of pay, time hours of work
        3. Auto insurance/reimbursement
        4. Dress code
        5. Insurance requirements
        6. Reporting illness
        7. Inservice meetings

II. Relationship of hospice care to other agencies and organizations
    A. Contractual agreements with other service providers
    B. Contractual agreements with subcontractors
    C. Community Resources

III. Discussion of referral sources
    A. Hospital: social worker, discharge planner/case manager, liaison
    B. Doctor
    C. Family
    D. Social agencies
    E. Staff

IV. Funding sources: discussion of the requirements of the funding sources
    A. Medicare
    B. Medicaid
    C. Blue Cross
    D. Private insurance
    E. Veterans Affairs
    F. Self Pay
        1. Full pay
        2. Part pay/fee adjustment
        3. No charge

V. Paperwork flow between clinical and office staff
    A. Instructions on use of day sheets
    B. Clinical charting and role of medical records

continues

VI. Individual responsibilities
    A. Job description _____
    B. Relationship to other members of staff _____
    C. Ethics _____
        1. Patients/families rights _____
        2. Confidentiality _____
VII. Explanation of the role of supervisor and the methods that will be used for evaluating performance and identifying needs
VIII. Policies and procedures
    A. Infection control: universal blood and body fluid precautions—OSHA's standards _____
    B. Safety/equipment management _____
    C. Quality assessment/improvement _____
    D. Advance directives/DNR _____
    E. Other relevant policies/procedures _____
IX. Terminal care/hospice _____
X. Home care specialty services
    A. IV team _____
    B. Maternal/child health _____
    C. Psychiatric _____
    D. Enterostomal therapy _____
    E. Incontinence management _____

I have read my job description and understand that I will be evaluated against these performance criteria.

Signature: _____

COP 418.56, 418.64

FORM 14

HOSPICE DISCHARGE CHECKLIST: INPATIENT

Patient: _____ Number: _____

	Complete	Incomplete	Correction Required By	Returned Init/Date
HOME CARE RECORD (right side)				
PMU 1				
Nursing Discharge Summary				
MFI				
Signed Interdisciplinary Care Plan Orders				
Physician Certificate of Terminal Illness (Medicare/MA only)				
Election of Hospice Benefit—Medicare only				
Hospice Program Consent for Care				
Release of Information Consent				
Authorization and Release Form				
Patient Bill of Rights and Responsibilities				
Medicare Secondary Payer Information				
INPATIENT RECORD (left side)				
Death Certificate				
Anatomical Donation				
Front Index Sheet				
Inpatient Face Sheet				
Physician Discharge Summary				
ER Record (if applicable)				
Progress Notes/Consults				

continues

	Complete	Incomplete	Correction Required By	Returned Init/Date
Clinical Notes (medications)				
Valuable Property Record				
Condition on Admission (if available)				
Vital Sign Records				
IV Records (if available)				
Written/Computer Orders				
Standards Documentation Flow Sheet				
IDG Patient Database				
Election of Hospice Benefit (copy)				
Hospice Program Consent for Care (copy)				
Release of Information Consent (copy)				
Living Will				
Authorization and Release Form (copy)				
Interdisciplinary Care Plan (orders)(copy)				
Referral for Services				
Nursing Assessment				
Braden/Nutrition Assessments				
MSW Assessment Form				
Volunteer Care Plan				
Volunteer Visit Records				

Checked by: _____ Date_____

COP 418.74

FORM 15

HOSPICE DISCHARGE CHECKLIST: ROUTINE AND INPATIENT RECORDS

Patient: _____ Number_____ Date Due_____ Start of Care _____

The discharge review indicated the following deficiencies. Please complete and return to Medical Records.

	Complete	Incomplete	Correction Required By	Returned Init/Date
RIGHT SIDE (Home Care)				
PMU 1				
Nursing Discharge Summary				
MFI Card				
Verbal Orders				
Interdisciplinary Care Plan (orders)				
Physician Certification of Terminal Illness (Medicare or MA benefit)				
Election of Hospice (Medicare benefit only)				
Hospice Program Patient Consent for Care				
Evaluation Forms—MSW, PT, OT				
HHA Plan of Care				
Volunteer Plan of Care				
Referral for Services (if no home care record)				
Authorization and Release Form (copy)				
Patient Bill of Rights and Responsibilities				
HHA Activity Records				
Progress Notes/Shingles				
NSG				
MSS				
PT				
OT				

continues

	Complete	Incomplete	Correction Required By	Returned Init/Date
ST				
Chaplain				
Volunteer				
Flow Sheets (all signed)				
Medication List (original)				
Nursing Assessment/Problem List				
LEFT SIDE (Hospital)				
Death Certificate				
Anatomical Donation				
Front Index Sheet				
Inpatient Face Sheet				
Physician Discharge Summary				
ER Record (if applicable)				
Progress Notes/Consults				
Clinical Notes (medications)				
Valuable Property Record				
Condition on Admission (if available)				
Vital Sign Records				
IV Records (if available)				
Written/Computer Orders				
Standards Documentation Flow Sheet				
IDG Patient Database				
Hospice Program IDG POC (copy)				
a) Any miscellaneous copies of hospice documents				
Hospice Volunteer POC				
Volunteer Activity Record				

Checked by: _____ Date_____

COP 418.74

FORM 16

HOSPICE DISCHARGE CHECKLIST: ROUTINE SERVICES

Patient: _____ Number_____ Date Due_____ Start of Care _____
The discharge review indicated the following deficiencies. Please complete and return to Medical Records.

	Complete	Incomplete	Correction Required By	Returned Init/Date
RIGHT SIDE				
PMU 1				
Nursing Discharge Summary				
Progress Notes/Shingles				
NSG				
MSS				
PT				
OT				
ST				
Chaplain				
Volunteer				
Flow Sheets (all signed)				
Medication List—original				
Nursing Assessment/Problem List				
LEFT SIDE				
MFI Card				
Verbal Orders				
Interdisciplinary Care Plan (orders)				
Physician Certification of Terminal Illness (Medicare or MA benefit only)				
Election of Hospice (Medicare benefit only)				
Hospice Program Patient Consent for Care				

continues

	Complete	Incomplete	Correction Required By	Returned Init/Date
Consent for Release of Information				
Evaluation Forms—MSW, PT, OT				
HHA Plan of Care				
Volunteer Plan of Care				
Referral for Services (if no home care record)				
Authorization and Release Form (copy from home care record)				
Patient Bill of Rights and Responsibilities				
HHA Activity Records				

Checked by: _____ Date_____

COP 418.74

FORM 17

HOSPICE HOME VISIT CONSENT FORM   Pt. # _____

1. Patient's Last Name:	First Name:	MI:	2. Health Insurance Claim #:

3. Patient's Address: (Street/City/State/ZIP Code)	4. Date of Birth:	5. Sex: M F

6. Hospice Name and Address (City and State)	7. Provider Number:

This consent form permits the fiscal intermediary medical review personnel to conduct home visits with you and/or your family members to ensure that quality care is provided and that Medicare payments for the services received are appropriate.

You and/or your family members have the right to refuse entry into your home at any time. Refusal to sign the home visit consent form or to permit entry into your home after consent is given will not affect payment for hospice services.

I understand the explanation described above and give my permission for home visits.

Beneficiary signature: _____ Date:_____

I understand the above explanation and choose not to allow a home visit.

Beneficiary signature: _____ Date:_____

_____
Signature of Hospice Representative

COP 418.62

FORM 18

HOSPICE MEDICARE BENEFIT REVOCATION

Patient Name: _____
Address: _____
_____

As a Medicare hospice beneficiary, I wish to revoke the election of Medicare coverage of hospice care for the remainder of benefit period #_____.

I understand that I am forfeiting the right to _____ days of hospice coverage in the current benefit period. Should I choose to reelect the Medicare Hospice Benefit at a later time, I retain the right to use _____ days in benefit period #_____, and, if applicable, _____ days in benefit period(s) #_____.

The benefit periods are as follows:
    First benefit period—90 days
    Second benefit period—90 days
    Unlimited benefit period—Renewed every 60 days

I direct this revocation to be effective on_____.

I understand that the Medicare health care benefits I waived to recieve hospice Medicare coverage will be resumed on the above-designated date.

_____ _____
Date   Signature of Beneficiary or Legal Representative

_____
Relationship of Legal Representative to Beneficiary

_____ _____
Date   Witness Signature

Note: Hospice revocation cannot be effective **prior** to the date this form is signed. A beneficiary may designate the effective date to be the same date as the signature date or a date in the future.

COP 418.28

FORM 19

HOSPICE VOLUNTEER BEREAVEMENT TRAINING SYLLABUS

This program will consist of lectures, videotapes, role playing, discussions, and group process conducted in 10 sessions by the director of volunteers.

- *Session 1:* Insight into the behavior patterns associated with loss, characteristics of grief, stages of loss, and various phenomena associated with grief.

- *Session 2:* Understanding grief and bereavement. Continuation of discussion of the grieving process, the rationale for bereavement support, and a sampling of successful interventions.

- *Session 3:* Patterns of grief process—a journey of changes.

- *Session 4:* Sidetracked or aborted grief that results in unresolved grief.

- *Session 5:* Effect on the immune system. Elaborates on how mourning can affect the griever's physical well-being.

- *Session 6:* How to cope with widowhood. Unguarded conversations from women who shared a common experience—widowhood.

- *Session 7:* Societal expectations and male grieving. The masculine mystique.

- *Session 8:* A child's understanding of death and a parent's grief when a child dies.

- *Session 9:* Rituals and traditions, religious beliefs related to death—different for everyone and every culture.

- *Session 10:* Benefits of support groups. Explanation of the bereavement program, initial assessment, periodic follow-up, and evaluation of risk factors. We offer a grief recovery program (12 sessions) in the spring and fall, plus individual counseling.

COP 418.70, 418.88

FORM 20

INTERDISCIPLINARY CARE PLAN

Patient Name: _____ Start of Care Date: _____
Address: _____ Medical Record No.: _____
_____ Provider No.: _____
Certification Period From: _____ To: _____

Medications (Dose/Freq/Route):
Standing Orders for General Hospice Kit Included. Administered by: _____

Compazine 25 MG PR Q6H PRN (3)
Compazine 10 MG PO Q6H PRN (3)
Roxanol (20 MG/ML) 5-10 MG SL Q2-3H PRN (3)
Levsin 0.125 MG SL Q4H PRN (5)
Haldol (2 MG/ML) 1 MG PO Q6H PRN (3)
Ativan 1 MG PO Q4H PRN (5)
Acetaminophen 650 MG PR Q4H PRN (3)

Principal Diagnosis: _____ DME/Supplies: _____
Other Diagnosis: _____ Hospital bed, BSC, Eggcrate Mattress,
Allergies: _____ Chux, Diapers, PRN
Mental Status: _____ Diet: _____
Activities Permitted: _____
Persons Participating in Care Plan Development: _____
Orders for Discipline and Treatments:
   Skilled Nursing: _____
   _____
   Home Health Aide: _____
   Social Service: _____
   Volunteers/Respite: _____
   Chaplain/Spiritual: _____
   Other: _____

PHYSICIAN CERTIFICATION: I/We certify/recertify that the above patient is terminally ill with a life expectancy of six months or less.

DO NOT RESUSCITATE: In the event of cardiac or respiratory arrest, CPR (cardiopulmonary resuscitation) measures will not be initiated.

The Hospice Interdisciplinary Care Plan is reviewed and revised at IDG meetings at least every two weeks.

_____   _____
Nurse's Signature   Date of Verbal Certification and Verbal
                                      Start of Care

_____   _____
Team Coordinator's Signature   Hospice Medical Director's Signature
Date Signed:_____   Date Signed: _____

_____
Attending Physician's Signature   Date Signed: _____
Physician Name:_____
Address: _____

COP 418.58

FORM 21

MSW COMPETENCY—IN-HOME EVALUATION

Employee Name: _____ Date of Visit: _____
Client Name: _____

                                                                                                                      Yes No N/A

Competency: Communication Skills for Dealing with Patients and Families
1. Communicates with client/family using professional verbal and nonverbal communication skills.
2. Discusses service to be provided and/or specific plans with patient prior to initiation of care.
3. Carries out home visit in organized, logical manner.
4. Informs client about each activity and receives his or her consent.
5. States purpose for next home visit.
6. Remains flexible during visit, adapting to the client/family needs.
7. Reviews tentative schedule of home visits.
8. Treats the patient with respect, dignity, professionalism.
9. Allows the patient to express feelings or concerns.
10. Includes significant others in the discussion (when appropriate).
11. Makes necessary accommodations when communicating with visually, hearing, or mentally impaired patient.
12. Demonstrates good listening skills.

Comments: _____

Competency: Safety and Infection Control
1. Handwashing done according to agency policy. (Washes hands before and after direct contact with patient.)
2. Observes precautions in handling blood or body fluids.

Comments: _____

Competency: Guidance and Client/Family Education
1. Involves client/family in care.
2. Uses language appropriate for client's level of understanding.
3. Counsels patients related to physical illness with consideration of patient's growth, development, and/or age.
4. Counsels patients unrelated to physical illness with consideration of patient's growth, development, and/or age.

Comments: _____

continues

	Yes	No	N/A

Competency: Care Consistent with Physician Plan of Treatment
1. Assesses client's ability to meet the medical and nursing requirements in regard to the home situation, financial resources, and availability of community resources.
2. Assesses client's ability to understand.
3. Assesses client's ability to follow medical recommendations.
4. Makes recommendations to client on use of selected community resources.

Comments: _____

Competency: Case Management
1. Involves client/family in care.
2. Communication includes discussion of other services.
3. Coordinates with other disciplines.
4. Communicates with and uses community resources.
5. Cooperates with other services in discharge planning.

Comments: _____

Competency: Assessment
1. Performs a psychosocial, emotional, and behavioral assessment cognizant of patient's age and diagnosis.
2. Possesses knowledge of stages of development through a patient's lifetime and uses this knowledge when assessing and counseling patients.

Comments: _____

Supervisor Signature/Date: _____

Employee Comments: _____
_____
_____

Employee Signature/Date: _____

COP 418.56, 418.64

FORM 22

NURSING COMPETENCY—IN-HOME EVALUATION
(Adult and Hospice Population)

Employee Name: _____ Date of Visit: _____
Client Number: _____

	Yes	No	N/A

Competency: Communication Skills for Dealing with Patients and Families
1. Communicates with client/family using professional verbal and nonverbal communication skills.
2. Discusses service to be provided and/or specific plans with patient prior to initiation of care.
3. Carries out home visit in organized, logical manner.
4. Informs client about each activity and receives his or her consent.
5. States purpose for next home visit.
6. Remains flexible during visit, adapting to the client/family needs.
7. Reviews tentative schedule of home visits for all disciplines involved in care.
8. Treats the patient with respect, dignity, professionalism.
9. Allows the adult patient to express feelings or concerns.
10. Includes significant others in the discussion (when appropriate).
11. Makes necessary accommodations when communicating with visually, hearing, or mentally impaired patient.
12. Demonstrates good listening skills.

Comments: _____

Competency: Safety and Infection Control
1. Handwashing done according to agency policy. (Washes hands before and after direct contact with patient.)
2. Nursing bag is properly cared for and protected.
3. Supplies and equipment maintained in the home and stored/utilized in appropriate manner.
4. Observes precautions in handling blood and body fluids.
5. Follows established protocol in handling and disposal of medical surgical supplies, needles and syringes, and infectious waste.
6. Assesses the safety of the home environment.

Comments: _____

Competency: Patient/Family Education
1. Uses language appropriate for client's level of understanding.
2. Follows logical sequence in instruction.
3. Demonstrates the care being taught.
4. Plans/carries out return demonstration.
5. Instructs on medication.

continues

	Yes	No	N/A

6. Educates the patient on home safety using age-specific educational materials.   ____ ____ ____

Comments: _____

Competency: Care Consistent with Physician Plan of Treatment
1. Carries out each medical order as described on plan.
2. Reports pertinent findings that need immediate report.
3. Urges client to seek medical care if indicated.
4. Checks medications to verify accuracy with plan of treatment.
5. Demonstrates technical skills needed to care for patient and carry out physician orders.
6. Demonstrates technical skills needed to provide infusion therapy, including restart, use of pumps, IV administration (IV/cardiac team).
7. Demonstrates knowledge of the cardiac care program and provides care consistent with the critical pathway and established protocols (IV/cardiac team).
8. Provides care consistent with the hospice plan of care (hospice only).

Comments: _____

Competency: Case Management
1. Uses all appropriate agency services.
2. Supervises HHA activities.
3. Uses community resources.
4. Uses appropriate patient education material.
5. Involves client/family in care.
6. Evaluates total plan of care with appropriate revisions, if indicated.
7. Performs discharge planning.

Comments: _____

Competency: Physical Assessment
1. Performs a physical assessment cognizant of patient's age and diagnosis.
2. Assesses the individual needs of the patient.
3. Integrates physical, social, and psychological factors when assessing the adult patient.
4. Completes a pain assessment and treats appropriately (hospice only).

Comments: _____

Supervisor Signature/Date: _____

Employee Comments: _____
_____
_____

Employee Signature/Date: _____

COP 418.56, 418.64

FORM 23

ORIENTATION PROGRAM

Name: _____ Date of Employment: _____

Position: _____

Date   Signature

DAY ONE

I. Orientation to agency structure/policies
   A. Introduction to Abington Memorial Hospital Home Care (AMHHC)
      1. Philosophy
         a. Self-care theory
         b. Community health standards
      2. Organizational structure
      3. Introduction to office personnel and facilities
      4. Sources of financial support
      5. Geographic area served
      6. Scope of services: Total program and services provided
   B. Medical policies and standing orders
   C. Nursing service policies
II. Personnel issues: Review and discussion
   A. Payroll procedure
   B. Schedule of pay, time, hours of work
   C. Auto insurance/reimbursement
   D. Dress code
   E. Insurance benefits
   F. Reporting illness
   G. Staff inservice meetings, outside activities, and advanced individual educational opportunities

DAY TWO
Field Observation with Staff

DAY THREE

I. Individual responsibilities
   A. Job description
   B. Standards
   C. Skilled care versus nonskilled care
II. Field assignments: Days and type of patient services
III. Criteria for admission of patients to home care
IV. Regulations governing home health aides
   A. Type of care provided
   B. Supervision of care

continues

Date   Signature

DAY FOUR

I. Relationship of nurse to other members of staff: RNs, PT, OT, ST, MSW, HHAs
    A. Individual responsibilities and relationships
    B. Coordination of services
    C. Role of nurse as case manager
II. Explanation of the role of supervisor and the methods used to evaluate performance and identify needs
III. Terminal care/hospice
IV. Home care specialty services
    A. IV team
    B. Maternal/child health
    C. Psychiatric
    D. Enterostomal therapy
    E. Incontinence management
V. Discussion of referral sources
    A. Hospital: Social worker, discharge planner
    B. Physician
    C. Family
    D. Social agencies
    E. Staff
VI. Relationship of AMHHC to other agencies and organizations
    A. Contractual agreement with homemaker/home health agencies
    B. Contractual agreement with other agencies
VII. Instructions on use of day sheets

DAY FIVE

I. Funding sources: Discussion of the requirements of the following funding sources:
    A. Medicare
    B. Medicaid
    C. Blue Cross
    D. HMO
    E. Private insurance
    F. Veterans Affairs
    G. Self-Pay
        1. Full pay
        2. Part pay/fee adjustment
        3. No charge
II. Discussion of the role of insurance case manager
III. Discussion of paper flow
IV. Discussion of all other forms used in the agency
V. Competency review and testing

continues

Date Signature

_____

DAY SIX

I. Discussion of professional ethics
    A. Patients/families' rights
    B. Confidentiality
II. Review of policies and procedures
    A. Infection control: Universal blood and body fluid precautions
    B. Safety (patient/staff)
    C. Equipment management
    D. Quality assessment/improvement
    E. Emergency preparedness
    F. Violence/neglect/abuse
    G. Advance directives/DNR
    H. Conflict of interest
    I. Other relevant policies/procedures
III. Community resources
IV. ATT Language line

DAY SEVEN

Introduction to Personal Computer

DAY EIGHT

I. Physical Assessment
II. High-volume disease entities
III. Agency for Health Care Policy and Research guidelines
    A. Pressure ulcers
    B. Urinary incontinence
    C. Pain
IV. Keystone Peer Review Organization standards

DAY NINE

Field observations with staff/clinical link daily visits

DAY TEN

Independent visits using clinical link

continues

Date   Signature

DAYS 11 THROUGH 14

Independent visits using clinical link   _____

DAYS 15, 18, 21, 22

Clinical link openings   _____

I have read my job description and understand that I will be evaluated against these performance criteria.

Employee Signature: _____

FORM 24
PAIN ASSESSMENT

PT. # _____ NAME _____ PG. _____

PARAMETERS/INTERVENTIONS	DATE	DATE	DATE	DATE	DATE	DATE	DATE	DATE	DATE	DATE	DATE	DATE
GOAL:												
ASSESSMENT												
Location of pain												
Type												
Intensity												
Onset-duration												
Associated symptoms												
Alleviated by												
Aggravated by												
Rest/activity patterns												
Mental status												
INSTRUCTION												
Side effects of analgesics: sedation, nausea, constipation												
Comfort measures												

continues

PARAMETERS/INTERVENTIONS	DATE	DATE	DATE	DATE	DATE	DATE	DATE	DATE	DATE	DATE	DATE	DATE
INTERVENTION AS INDICATED												
Pain Control: Method												
Med dose												
Frequency												
Relief												
Breakthrough pain												
RN signature (initials)												
Intensity Scale (0–5 Scale)												
0 = No Pain; 5 = Excruciating Pain												

C = Care; D = Disc; E = Eval; N = Narrative; DNA = Does Not Apply; NA = Not Assessed; IB = Instr. Begun; IC = Instr. Contd.; S = Supvsn.; U = Unchgd.; + = Yes; – = No

COP 418.82

FORM 25

PATIENT CONSENT FOR CARE

I, _____, hereby consent to admission to Abington Memorial Hospital
   (Print Patient's Name)
Home Care Hospice Program.

I acknowledge and consent to the following:

1. I understand Abington Memorial Hospital Home Care Hospice's goal is not to cure my terminal illness. The program staff, including volunteers, will work to reduce symptoms such as pain and nausea. Hospice staff will also provide emotional support and spiritual support (when requested) to me and my family and/or primary care person in my home.

2. Since the focus of hospice is to neither prolong life nor hasten death, I understand that hospice will not prolong my life by performing CPR (cardiopulmonary resuscitation) unless otherwise directed to do so.

3. I understand that _____ will be considered my primary care person. This
                              (Name)
means he/she will be mainly responsible for looking after me in my home. He/she is designated to make decisions on my behalf in the event I am unable to communicate them.

   I understand that if I live alone, I agree to abide by the hospice's recommendations for the safe delivery of care.

4. I understand that care is intermittent and will be provided by scheduled appointments, but that assistance is available 24 hours a day. The hospice service number is (____)____-_____.

5. Charges for household and support services such as companions and housekeeping are not covered by most health plans. Should such services be necessary, I am responsible for payment.

6. I understand that as long as I am enrolled in this hospice program, a team of caregivers will manage my care whether I am being cared for in my home or
   - at Abington Memorial Hospital for short-term management of acute symptoms
   - at a contract skilled nursing facility for short-term respite.

7. I understand that the durable medical equipment necessary for pain and symptom control will be provided for me through contract medical equipment companies. Medication for pain and symptom control is provided through contract pharmacies.

8. I understand that the hospice medical record will contain information about me, my family, and/or my primary care person. Every effort will be made to keep this information confidential. Information about me will be exchanged with my family.

9. I understand that if I am to receive full benefits of hospice care, it is important for me to make my needs and concerns known to the hospice staff. I will actively participate in plans for my care.

10. I authorize the care to begin on: _____

_____
Date   Signature of Patient or Legal Representative

_____
Date   Signature of Primary Care Person

_____
Date   Witness Signature

COP 418.62

FORM 26

PHYSICIAN CERTIFICATION/RECERTIFICATION OF TERMINAL ILLNESS

Patient Name: _____ Medical Record No.: _____

CERTIFICATION STATEMENT—FIRST BENEFIT PERIOD (90 DAYS)

Certification Period From: _____ To: _____
We (or I) certify that to the best of our (my) knowledge _____
 (Patient's Name)
is terminally ill with _____ and has a life expectancy of six (6) months or less.

_____
Hospice Medical Director or Designee   Date Signed

_____
Attending Physician   Date Signed

RECERTIFICATION STATEMENT—SECOND BENEFIT PERIOD (90 DAYS)

Certification Period From: _____ To: _____
I recertify that to the best of my knowledge the above patient is still considered terminally ill with _____ and has a life expectancy of six (6) months or less.

_____
Hospice Medical Director or Designee   Date Signed

RECERTIFICATION STATEMENT—UNLIMITED BENEFIT PERIOD (RENEWED EVERY 60 DAYS)

Certification Period From: _____ To: _____
I recertify that to the best of my knowledge the above patient is still considered terminally ill with _____ and has a life expectancy of six (6) months or less.

_____
Hospice Medical Director or Designee   Date Signed

COP 418.22

FORM 27

PLAN OF CARE FOR INPATIENT RESPITE

Patient Name: _____ Admission Date: _____

Address: _____ Facility Name: _____

Telephone: _____ Patient Diagnosis: _____

Reason for Transfer: _____

Description of patient's general condition (including vs/range): _____

              Needs   Bowel incontinence: Yes___ No___
ADL   Indep. Asst. Unable   Special regimen: _____
Turn/sit   Urinary incontinence: Yes___ No___
Bed to Chair   Special regimen: _____
Walking   Primary caregiver in home: _____
With walker   Religion: _____
With crutches   Advance Directive: _____
With cane
Stairs   Patient Mental Status   Caregiver status & ability
Bathe self   Good _____   Good _____
Dress self   Fair _____   Fair _____
Feed self   Poor _____   Poor _____
Mouth care
Shave   Home Environment   Equipment used in home:
To bathroom   Good _____   _____
Commode   Fair _____   _____
Bedpan/urinal   Poor _____   Funeral Home_____

Medications (Dose/Freq/Route):
_____
_____

Physicians orders for service & treatments (Please access RN on call at _____
for questions/problem):
_____
_____
_____
_____

Physician Certification: I/we certify that the above patient is terminally ill with a life expectancy of 6 months or less. **DO NOT RESUSCITATE:** In the event of cardiac or respiratory arrest, CPR (cardiopulmonary resuscitation) measures will not be initiated.

Physician's Signature: _____

Hospice Coordinator's Signature: _____

Signature of Person Completing Form: _____ Date: _____

COP 418.56(e)

FORM 28

QUALITY ASSURANCE QUARTERLY RECORD REVIEW
NURSING (HOSPICE)

Client Name: _____   Date of Review: _____

Client Case No.: _____   Present Quarter: _____

Primary Nurse Name: _____   Months Included: _____

Status of Record: Active _____
    Discharged _____   _____
                                                                   Signature of Reviewer

Services Involved

	Yes	No	N/A	Comments
I. ASSESSMENT				
A. Does the clinical record include assessment of physical, psychosocial, spiritual (including religious orientation), and environmental needs of patient/family?				
B. Was the nursing assessment form updated upon each new plan of treatment, past each hospitalization, or with transfer to benefit? (Include problem list.)				
C. Were nursing diagnoses based on assessment factors?				
D. Did the primary nurse select the correct patient group on admission?				
E. If the patient's status changed, was the patient group changed accordingly?				
II. PLANNING				
A. Were client goals stated on nursing assessment and flowsheets?				
B. Were the nursing parameters specific to the identified nursing diagnosis/problem?				
C. Was the plan of treatment (POT) current and signed by the primary physician and medical director?				
D. Was the POT completed in accordance with agency policy?				
1. Does the POT include assessment and identify management of discomfort and symptom relief?				

continues

		Yes	No	N/A	Comments
	2. Does POT include assessment of caregiver's respite needs and respite care?				
E.	Were signed verbal orders obtained to cover any change in the plan of treatment (including DME and supplies)?				
F.	Was the interdisciplinary group plan of care (as noted in team conference notes) reviewed and revised at least q2 weeks?				
III. IMPLEMENTATION					
A.	Was the frequency of nursing visits based on the assessment of the client's needs?				
B.	Was the service provided consistent with the care plan?				
C.	Does the record contain evidence that the applicable subobjectives in the patient classification/objectives system were being acted upon?				
D.	Does the record contain evidence that symptom management and comfort care needs were addressed and acted upon?				
E.	Did the nurse request consultative services of other disciplines when needed? (Describe.)				
F.	Did the nurse regularly supervise the performance of the HHA/LPN?				
G.	HHA consistent with client's needs?				
H.	Did the nurse demonstrate evidence of his/her coordination of all services?				
I.	Did the nurse hold conferences/joint visits with other disciplines when appropriate?				
J.	Did the nurse notify the physician/ other team members of any significant changes in the client's status?				
K.	Were service reports legible, dated, and signed?				
L.	Did service reports include:				
	1. Adequate information regarding the client's current condition?				
	2. Specific treatments/instructions given? (including 24 hr. emergency access)				

continues

	Yes	No	N/A	Comments
3. The date of the next visit?				
M. Were the following forms present and updated according to agency protocol:				
1. Authorization and Release Form? (copies)				
2. Bill of Rights? (copies)				
3. HHA plan of care?				
4. Medicare termination letter?				
N. Does the record contain evidence that medications were checked for significant side effects and indications?				
O. Were interdisciplinary group conferences documented including all applicable disciplines and plan for next week?				
P. Were the following forms present and completed according to agency policy?				
1. Election of Hospice Medicare Benefit—Informed Consent (for each benefit period)				
2. Hospice Program Patient Consent for care				
3. Physician Certification of Terminal Illness—signed by both physicians (Medicare and MA only)				
4. Change or Revocation of Hospice				
IV. EVALUATION				
A. Were patient/family responses to nursing intervention documented?				
1. Does the record reflect the patient/family received necessary preparation for death?				
B. Were necessary modifications in the care plan made based on the nurse's evaluation?				
C. If patient discharged from nursing service:				
1. Was discharge a logical development of the care plan and client goals?				

continues

		Yes	No	N/A	Comments
	2. Does the record contain a description of the patient/family change in knowledge, understanding, and/or behavior as the result of the nurse's intervention?				
	3. Was there evidence of the client's goals having been met?				
	4. Was discharge summary present and accurately completed?				
	5. Were the nursing diagnoses on the discharge computer summary consistent with those on the problem list?				
	6. Were the service codes (group number and goal attainment) listed on the discharge computer summary consistent with the evidence found in the record?				
	7. Was the physician notified of client's discharge?				
D.	Patient discharge reason:				
	1. Death				
	2. Remission/improved				
	3. Moved out of area				
	4. Other				
E.	If discharged from service was due to death, is there documentation of a final team conference reflecting a referral for bereavement services?				
V. UTILIZATION REVIEW					
A.	80% of routine care was delivered at home.				
B.	20% or less was delivered in inpatient setting.				
C.	Change in level of care was implemented when needed:				
	1. Acute care at AMH for a symptom that could not be managed at home.				
	2. Respite care at contract nursing home for 5 days or less.				

continues

	Yes	No	N/A	Comments
3. Continuous RN/LPN care during periods of crises.				
D. Was the length of service greater than 210 days?				
E. In the opinion of the reviewer, were services:				
1. Appropriately utilized?				
2. Overutilized?				
3. Underutilized?				

COP 418.66

FORM 29

RESOURCE LIST—RELIGIOUS GROUPS

List local religious organizations, contact persons, and telephone numbers. For example:

ARMENIAN:

_____

_____

BUDDHIST:

_____

_____

FIRST CHURCH OF CHRIST SCIENTIST:

_____

_____

JEHOVAH'S WITNESS:

_____

_____

JEWISH

  Reform: _____

  Conservative: _____

SEVENTH DAY ADVENTIST:

_____

_____

UNITARIAN-UNIVERSALIST:

_____

_____

LOCAL CHURCHES

Baptist:

_____

_____

Brethren:

_____

_____

continues

Catholic:
_____
_____

Episcopal:
_____
_____

Friends:
_____
_____

Lutheran:
_____
_____

Presbyterian:
_____
_____

United Methodist:
_____
_____

Other:
_____
_____

COP 418.70(f), 418.88

FORM 30

RESOURCE LIST—SUGGESTED READINGS ON DEATH, DYING, BEREAVEMENT

Angel, M.D. 1987. *The orphaned adult: Confronting the death of a parent.* New York: Insight Books.

Presented here is a thoughtful discussion of the processes of adult orphanhood and practical as well as philosophical issues from personal experiences to general themes of mortality, mourning, and permanent influences of parents.

Benton, R. 1978. *Death and dying: Principles and practices in patient care.* New York: Van Nostrand Reinhold.

As its title indicates, this volume covers the topic in depth for the health professional and the mourning principals.

Bluebond-Langner, M. 1978. *The private worlds of dying children.* Princeton, NJ: Princeton University Press.

The observations in this doctoral dissertation suggest that dying children are more aware of what is going on in their lives than they are given credit for by parents, physicians, nurses, and social scientists, who regard them as passive recipients of adult actions.

Buckman, R. 1988. *I don't know what to say, how to help and support someone who is dying.* Toronto: Key Porter Books.

Very well-organized, comprehensive volume written specifically for family and friends of a dying person. Covers all aspects.

Burgess, J.K. 1988. *The single again man.* Lexington, MA: D.C. Heath & Co.

A very helpful book to assist grieving men overcome grief and learn to live again. It is also the author's aim to educate society that men need the same sympathy and emotional support offered women.

Caine, L. 1988. *Being a widow: A helpful guide to the problems of being a widow.* New York: William Morrow.

A self-help book full of practical advice and words of wisdom. Answers to many questions that a widow faces.

Caine, L. 1978. *Lifelines.* New York: Doubleday.

Practical advice for women who have to cope with life alone, how author dealt with her own emotional, financial, and physical problems since the death of her husband.

Caine, L. 1974. *Widow.* New York: William Morrow.

Personal experiences after death of husband. Her story is a candid and moving account that can help and enlighten all.

Carroll, D. 1985. *Living with dying: A loving guide for family and close friends.* New York: McGraw-Hill.

A comprehensive, easy-to-read, practical guide to dying. It covers a wide range of topics from grieving to care at home, hospice and funeral arrangements.

continues

Cohn, J. 1987. *I had a friend named Peter: Talking to children about the death of a friend.* New York: William Morrow.

    Author presents guidelines that answer questions that parents and teachers may have about talking to children about death.

Cuming, P. 1981. *Widow's walk: A personal journey through loss, fear, anger, and love.* New York: Crown.

    Personal account of a young widow's first year's journey with the fears and frustration of widowhood.

Cutter, F. 1974. *Coming to terms with death: How to face the inevitable with wisdom and dignity.* Chicago: Nelson Hall.

    The author's hope is that "this book will provide readers with help in how to prepare for death of others and to help the dying retain dignity."

Doka, K. 1989. *Disenfranchised grief: Recognizing hidden sorrow.* New York: D.C. Heath & Co.

    This book helps those whose loss is not openly or socially acknowledged and who are therefore deprived of the catharsis that shared grief brings.

Donnelly, K.F. 1988. *Recovering from the loss of a sibling.* New York: Dodd Mead.

    This book provides a catharsis in the sharing of experiences. Part of the getting well process is going through the pain of grief.

Donnelly, K.F. 1982. *Recovering from the loss of a child.* New York: Macmillan.

    An invaluable resource for bereaved parents and other survivors and an aid for those working in helping professions. Part II describes the growing network of self-help associations that provide family support.

Ginsberg, G.D. 1987. *To live again: Rebuilding your life after you've become a widow.* Los Angeles: Jeremy P. Tarcher.

    Discusses in very readable language the needs of average middle-aged widows. A book for those coping with the death of a loved one.

Graham, V. 1988. *Life after Harry: My adventures in widowhood.* New York: Simon & Schuster.

    The actress and lecturer presents her account of the "struggles of widowhood." "Life after Harry, or Tom, or Dick can be a satisfying and stimulating time."

Grollman, E., ed. 1967. *Explaining death to children.* Boston: Beacon Press.

    Several contributors (chapters) write on the subject of the title.

Hamilton, M., and H.F. Reid. 1980. *A hospice handbook: A new way to care for the dying.* Grand Rapids, MI: William B. Erdman's Publishing Co.

    Hospice is part of a movement to humanize the way medical care is given. The movement has focused on the beginning as well as the end of life. The book explains that hospice, while meeting medical needs, also provides emotional and spiritual support and understanding for those facing death.

Hughes, T.E., and D. Klein. 1983. *A family guide to estate planning, funeral arrangements, and settling an estate after death.* New York: Charles Scribner's Sons.

    This volume explains how estate planning makes the after death period easier for survivors and allows them to proceed with confidence because they are informed.

continues

Jackson, E. 1965. *Telling a child about death*. New York: Hawthorne.
　How to honestly answer questions children ask when facing the facts of death and bereavement.

Jackson, E. 1957. *Understanding grief: Its roots, dynames, and treatment*. Nashville, TN: Abington Press.
　A comprehensive study of grief and methods of counseling the grief-stricken.

Jewett, C. 1982. *Helping children cope with separation and loss*. Cambridge, MA: Harvard Common Press.
　The author has developed simple techniques that any adult can use to help children through grief. Describes stages of mourning and expected behavior.

Johnson, S. 1977. *First person singular: Living the good life alone*. New York: Lippincott-Raven Publishers.
　The author's purpose is to show single adults in a couple oriented culture how to overcome the problems and fulfill the promise of living in the first person singular.

Kirsch, C. 1981. *A survivor's manual to contingency planning: Wills, trusts, guidelines to guardians, getting through probate, taxes, life insurance, maintaining emotional stability, protection from reckless spending, living on fixed income, reconciling family differences, avoiding con artists*. New York: Doubleday.
　The complete title says it all.

Kohn. J.B. 1978. *The Widower*. Boston: Beacon Press.
　Deals specifically with the special emotional and practical problems of the widower.

Kubler-Ross, E. 1983. *On children and death*. New York: Macmillan.
　The author confronts difficulties faced by parents of dying children and offers the practical help needed at this critical time.

Kubler-Ross, E. 1978. *To live until we say goodbye*. Englewood Cliffs, NJ: Prentice Hall.
　The beautiful black and white photos and the author's text illustrate what can and will happen to human beings, young and old, when they are in the process of being destroyed by a malignant growth but are able to emerge with a sense of peace and freedom.

Kubler-Ross, E. 1975. *Death, the final stage of growth*. Englewood Cliffs, NJ: Prentice Hall.
　The author has gathered different views on the subject of death that guide the reader in search for the meaning of life and death.

Kubler-Ross, E. 1974. *Questions and answers on death and dying*. New York: Macmillan.
　This sequel to *On Death and Dying* (1969) consists of the most frequently asked questions and the author's responses arranged to help the readers faced with like situations.

Kubler-Ross, E. 1969. *On death and dying*. New York: Macmillan.
　Written in non-technical language, this book offers a humane approach to relieving the psychological suffering of the terminally ill. It shows how the dying can be helped to meet their death in peace and dignity.

LeShan, E. 1976. *Learning to say good-by: When a parent dies*. New York: Macmillan.
　In simple language, the author discusses the questions, fears, and fantasies children have about parents who have died and people still alive.

continues

Loewinsoh, R.J. 1979. *Survival handbook for widows (and for relatives and friends who want to understand)*. Chicago: Follett.

    Empathetic and helpful to the needs of widows and widowers.

Marshall, M.L. 1988. *The re-mating game: Dating and relating in middle age*. Whitehall, VA: Betterway Publications.

    Down-to-earth advice and suggestions for those (widows and widowers included) who are reentering the dating scene.

Maxwell, K. 1988. *No lifetime guarantee: Dealing with the details of death*. Whitehall, VA: Betterway Publications.

    A comprehensive handbook providing information, explanations, and options relating to death. Includes alternatives for the dying (hospice), living wills, and organ donation and goes on from there with funeral arrangements, wills and probate, teaming up with a professional advisor, Social Security, real estate, and taxes.

Mooney, E.C. 1981. *Alone: Surviving as a widow*. New York: G.P. Putnam's Sons.

    One woman's story about being widowed, about how to gain courage and triumph over social mores that say we must be part of a couple. How to endure aloneness.

Morgan, E. 1988. *Dealing creatively with death: A manual of death, education, and simple education*. 11th ed. Burnsville, NC: Celo Press.

    As the word *manual* implies, this small encyclopedia covers all aspects of death and dying. Also included are appendices listing bibliographies, organizations, and services.

Munley, A. 1983. *The hospice alternative: A new context for death and dying*. New York: Basic Books.

    A definitive work on this innovative and important system for providing humane care and support to the dying and their families.

Myers, E. 1986. *When parents die: A guide for adults*. New York: Viking.

    This book can be recommended to any adult dealing with death or serious illness of a parent. Enormously helpful including an excellent Further Reading List.

Neeld, E.H., 1990. *Seven choices: Taking the steps to a new life after losing someone you love*. New York: Potter.

    The book identifies the seven major phases of grief as the author sees them and explains how understanding them can help readers cope with loss.

Nudel, A.R. 1986. *Starting over: Help for young widows and widowers*. New York: Dodd Mead.

    A guide for the younger widowed person, a book of advice and comfort.

Peck, R., and C. Stefanics. 1987. *Learning to say goodbye: Dealing with death and dying*. Muncie, IN: Accelerated Development.

    Features humanistic approach to death and dying. Provides information for dealing with needs of the triad in health care system: the patient, the family, and the staff.

Pike, M.V., and J. Armstrong. 1980–81. *A time to mourn: Customs and rites—expressions of grief in nineteenth century America*. New York: Museums of Stony Brook.

    A museum catalog, a result of National Endowment for the Humanities. The text and photos express death, grief, and mourning in nineteenth-century America.

continues

Pincus, L. 1974. *Death and the family: The importance of mourning.* New York: Pantheon.
Telling her own story and those of others, the author focuses on the elements of bereavement useful for the bereaved and those who care for them to understand. Also valuable for those who would rather face the harsh realities of life than deny them.

Rando, T.A. 1991. *Grieving: How to go on living when someone you love dies.* Lexington, MA: D.C. Heath & Co.
A very comprehensive book to help the bereaved and those who care for them. Valuable, clear advice on dealing with many problems, practical and emotional, shared by mourners.

Rosen, H. 1988. *Unspoken grief: Coping with childhood sibling loss.* Lexington, MA: D.C. Heath & Co.
Very comprehensive study of sibling loss.

Rudolph, M. 1978. *Should the children know? Encounters with death in the lives of children.* New York: Schocken Books.
Explains how the very young can be taught about death at school and at home through books, care of plants and animals, and direct experiences with human death.

Schiff, H.S. 1977. *The Bereaved Parent.* New York: Crown.
The author, whose 10-year-old son died, offers comfort and compassion, guiding other parents through their feelings of grief, guilt, and hopelessness.

Schuh, N. 1978. *After winter, spring.* Plainfield, NJ: Logos International.
A year-long personal account, a daily journal following the death of the author's husband. A moving study on the grieving process.

Simpson, M.A. 1979. *The facts of death: A complete guide for being prepared.* Englewood Cliffs, NJ: Prentice Hall.
The author offers a complete guide for "being prepared" to face one's own death, to talk with the dying, to comfort the bereaved, and to handle funeral arrangements, wills, and taxes, etc.

Stein, S.B. 1974. *About dying: An open family book for parents and children together.* New York: Walker and Co.
Using black and white photos and a divided text, one for the adult and one for the child, creates a shared experience discussing death.

Sternberg, F., and B. Sternberg. 1980. *If I die and when I do.* Englewood Cliffs, NJ: Prentice Hall.
The authors capture the spirit of young people as they explore death and life. The main subject, while death, is really about life.

Stoddard, S. 1978. *The hospice movement: A better way of caring for the dying.*
How the hospice approach helps terminally ill patients face death without pain or fear. Why and how hospices work.

Taves, I. 1981. *The widows guide.* New York: Schocken Books.
As the title indicates, this volume offers practical advice on how to deal with grief, stress, health, children, family, work, and getting back into the world.

Taves, I. 1974. *Love must not be wasted: When sorrow comes, take it gently by the hand.* New York: Crowell.
The author explores the subject of bereavement and grief.

continues

Temes, R. 1977. *Living with an empty chair: A guide through grief.* Amherst, MA: Mandella Publishing Co.

    This book addresses those who are not dying but must continue to live even when a loved one is dead. A helpful dissertation for the recently bereaved, the professional (social worker, psychologist), physician, funeral director, neighbor, friend.

Upson, N. 1986. *When someone you love is dying.* New York: Simon & Schuster.

    A helpful guide for those who are the supporting cast in the last act of a loved one's life.

Viorst, J. 1986. *Necessary losses.* New York: Simon & Schuster.

    Writing about the human condition, the author demonstrates what is given up in order to grow. She helps the reader understand and deal with "necessary losses."

Weizman, S.G., and P. Kamm. 1987. *About mourning: Support and guidance for the beareaved.* New York: Human Sciences Press.

    A book for the bereaved offering comfort and support. The well-organized chapters cover all aspects of death, grief, and mourning.

Wentzel, K.B. 1981. *To those who need it most, hospice means hope.* Boston: Charles River Books.

    Extensive information about the hospice program. Helpful for families in which someone has a terminal illness and could benefit from the program.

COP 418.88

FORM 31

SPIRITUAL/RELIGIOUS ASSESSMENT

Name: _____ Record Number: _____

Family Members: _____ Relationship: _____

_____

_____

Church or Religious Affiliation: _____

_____

Relationship with church or synagogue? _____

_____

Does patient or family wish contact with pastor/priest/rabbi from hospice team?_____

Would the patient and/or family members wish to have Sacraments brought to the home? _____

Any special feelings expressed toward religion? _____

_____

Presence of religious symbols? _____

Is the patient/family open to receiving prayer from the chaplain? _____

Patient's/caregiver's spiritual or religious concerns: _____

_____

What is the patient's attitude/response to pain? _____

_____

Feelings/conditions expressed by the patient: _____

_____

Goals:

Plans:

Signature: _____ Date:_____

COP 418.70(f), 418.88(c)

FORM 32

THERAPY COMPETENCY IN-HOME EVALUATION

Employee Name: _____ Date of Visit: _____

Client Name: _____

	Yes	No	N/A

Competency: Communication Skills for Dealing with Patients and Families
1. Communicates with client/family using professional verbal and non-verbal communication skills.
2. Discusses service to be provided and/or specific plans with patient prior to initiation of care.
3. Carries out home visit in organized, logical manner.
4. Informs client about each activity and receives his/her consent.
5. States purpose for next home visit/schedules next visit.
6. Remains flexible during visit, adapting to the client/family needs.
7. Reviews tentative schedule of home visits.
8. Treats the patient with respect, dignity, and professionalism.
9. Allows the patient to express feelings or concerns.
10. Includes significant others in the discussion.
11. Makes necessary accommodations when communicating with visually, hearing, or mentally impaired patient.

Comments: _____

Competency: Safety and Infection Control
1. Handwashing done according to policy. (Washes hands before and after direct contact with patient.)
2. Supplies and equipment maintained in the home and stored/utilized in appropriate manner.
3. Observes precautions in handling blood or bodily fluids.
4. Assesses the safety of the home environment.

Comments: _____

Competency: Patient/Family Education
1. Uses language appropriate for client's level of understanding.
2. Uses logical sequence in instruction.
3. Demonstrates care being taught.
4. Plans or carries out return demonstration.
5. Provides written instructions as needed.

Comments: _____

continues

	Yes	No	N/A

Competency: Care Consistent with Physician Plan of Treatment
1. Carries out each medical order as described on POT.
2. Makes observations/assessments in accordance with diagnosis and client needs.
3. Reports pertinent findings to physician.
4. Urges client to seek medical care if indicated.

Comments: _____

Competency: Case Management
1. Involves client/family in care.
2. Coordinates plan of care, with appropriate revisions, with nurse case manager.
3. Performs discharge planning.

Comments: _____

Competency: Basic Skills (Physical Therapist only)
1. Gait training (walker, quad cane, straight cane, crutches, forearm crutches, platform crutches).
2. Transfer training (from all elevations).
3. Active range of motion exercises.
4. Passive range of motion exercises.
5. Active-assistive range of motion exercises.

Comments: _____

Competency: Basic Skills (Occupational Therapist only)
1. Functional transfer training.
2. Wheelchair mobility.
3. Adaptive equipment.
4. Self-care training.
5. Therapeutic exercise.
6. Body mechanics.

Comments: _____

_____

Supervisor Signature/Date: _____

Employee Comments: _____

_____

Employee Signature/Date: _____

COP 418.56

FORM 33

VOLUNTEER ASSESSMENT AND PLAN: INPATIENT UNIT

Patient No.: _____   Patient Name: _____

Age: _____   Room Number: _____

Diagnosis: _____

Functional limitations/clinical considerations: _____

_____

_____

_____

Mental Status: _____

_____

Special Interests/Diversions/Hobbies: _____

VOLUNTEER ASSIGNMENT

If area of need is identified by a checkmark, service may be provided when requested by the patient/family. If box is *not* checked, that service cannot be provided unless it is first authorized by the volunteer director, hospice case manager, or the patient's primary nurse.

Patient Care Needs Requiring Volunteer Assistance:

_____	Meals/feeding/fluids	_____
_____	Ambulation	_____
_____	Transfers	_____
_____	Toileting	_____
_____	Positioning	_____
_____	Diversional activities	_____
_____	Companionship	_____
_____	Mouth care	Every hour with cold water and green swabs; petroleum to lips
_____	Skin care	Lotion to elbows, hands, heels, and feet every four hours
_____	Other	_____

Significant Family Members, Family Considerations: _____

_____

Volunteer Goals: _____

Signature: _____   Date: _____

COP 418.70

FORM 34

VOLUNTEER TRAINING PROGRAM SYLLABUS

Session 1: *Introduction*—Orientation; history of hospice movement and goals of hospice program.

Process Issues—Verbal communications; the volunteer's personal interactions with the patient and family. Active listening; content and affect responses.

Session 2: *Primary Care Issues*—The hospice RN, nursing skills, nursing procedures for hospice patients; discussion of pain and symptom control; patient care and comfort; terminality, physical change, and problems.

Session 3: *Process Issues*—Spiritual support communication skills; working through patients' and families' spiritual feelings; liaison role between patients' and families' clergy and hospice team.

Session 4: *Process Issues*—Sociological considerations; communication skills; working through patients' and families' emotional feelings; liaison role between patients and hospice team; social worker's involvement with families and support system.

Session 5: *OSHA Training* (Occupational Safety and Health Administration)—Training that includes bloodborne pathogens information required of all home care volunteers.

Competency Performance and Evaluation—Handwashing with waterless cleansing agent. Donning and removal of gloves.

Demonstration—Skills demonstrated and practiced by volunteers; assisting patients with physical limitations.

Session 6: *Process Issues*—The ethics and values of team process; family issues; respect for patient/family; ethical issues such as confidentiality and patient/family rights. Panel discussion with experienced volunteers. The role of volunteers in providing care and comfort.

Process Issues—Bereavement support programs; initial assessment; periodic follow-up; evaluation of risk factors, memorial service, the values of team process; overview of bereavement training program.

Practicum—Individual assignment to cover home and hospice unit in AMH visit.

COP 418.70

PART III

List of Medicare Conditions of Participation Cross-References

Medicare COP		Handbook of Hospice Policies and Procedures
Subpart B—Eligibility, Election, and Duration of Benefits		
418.20	Eligibility requirements	1:21
418.21	Duration of hospice care coverage—Election periods	1:21; Form 10
418.22	Certification of terminal illness	Form 26 and 27
418.24	Election of hospice care	1:21
418.28	Revoking the election of hospice care	1:21; Form 18
418.30	Change of designated hospice	Form 6
Subpart C—Conditions of Participation, General Provisions, and Administration		
418.50	Conditions of Participation—General Provisions	1:15
418.52	Condition of Participation—Governing Body	1:25
418.54	Condition of Participation—Medical Director	1:43
418.56	Condition of Participation—Professional Management	1:40, 1:46, 1:53, 1:63
418.58	Condition of Participation—Plan of care	1:38, 1:43
418.60	Condition of Participation—Continuation of Care	1:17
418.62	Condition of Participation—Informed Consent	1:05; Form 10
418.64	Condition of Participation—Inservice Training	1:64
418.66	Condition of Participation—Quality Assurance	1:57
418.68	Condition of Participation—Interdisciplinary Group	1:36, 1:37, 1:38
418.70	Condition of Participation—Volunteers	1:71, 1:72
418.72	Condition of Participation—Licensure	1:15
418.74	Condition of Participation—Central Clinical Records	1:10

Medicare COP		Handbook of Hospice Policies and Procedures
Subpart D—Conditions of Participation: Core Services		
418.80	Condition of Participation—Furnishing of Core Services	1:15
418.82	Condition of Participation—Nursing Services	1:07, 1:16, 1:45
418.83	Nursing services—Waiver of requirements that substantially all nursing services be routinely provided directly by a hospice.	1:15
418.84	Condition of Participation—Medical Social Services	1:62
418.86	Condition of Participation—Physician Services	1:43
418.88	Condition of Participation—Counseling Services	1:15
Subpart E—Conditions of Participation: Other Services		
418.90	Condition of Participation—Furnishing of Other Services	1:46, 1:53, 1:63
418.92	Condition of Participation—Physical Therapy, Occupational Therapy, and Speech-Language Pathology	1:46, 1:53, 1:63
418.94	Condition of Participation—Home Health Aides and Homemaker Services	1:27
418.96	Condition of Participation—Medical Supplies	1:15, 1:26
418.98	Condition of Participation—Short-Term Inpatient Care	1:03
418.100	Condition of Participation for Freestanding Hospices Providing Inpatient Care Directly	n/a to AMH

APPENDIX A

Federal Register Material

Appendix A includes selected Federal Registers that reference the Medicare Hospice program. The 1983, 1984, 1987, and 1990 Federal Registers provide updates to the program. Transmittal No. A 98-27 contains the hospice provisions enacted by the Balanced Budget Act of 1997. Please reference the most recent publications for current information.

PART VII

DEPARTMENT OF HEALTH AND HUMAN SERVICES

Health Care Financing Administration
Medicare Program; Hospice Care; Final Rule

PART 408—MEDICARE ELIGIBILITY AND ENTITLEMENT

The authority citation for Part 408 reads as follows:
Authority: Secs. 202 (t) and (u), 226, 226A, 1102, 1811 and 1818 of the Social Security Act (42 U.S.C. 402 (t) and (u), 426, 426-1, 1302, 1395c, 1395i-2. Section 103 of Publ. L. 89-97 (42 U.S.C 426a)).

F. Part 408 is amended as follows: Section 408.2 is revised to read as follows:

§ 408.2 Scope.

This subpart specifies the conditions of eligibility for hospital insurance and sets forth certain specific conditions that affect entitlement to benefits. Hospital insurance is authorized under Part A 1 of 2 Title XVIII and is also referred to as Medicare Part A. It includes inpatient hospital care, posthospital skilled nursing facility care, posthospital home health services, and hospice care.

PART 409—MEDICARE BENEFITS, LIMITATIONS, AND EXCLUSIONS

The authority citation for Part 409 reads as follows:
Authority: Secs. 1102, 1812, 1813, 1814, 1861, 1866, 1871, 1881, and 1883 of the Social Security Act (42 U.S.C. 1302, 1395d, 1395e, 1395f, 1395x, 1395cc, 1395hh, 1395rr, and 1395tt).

G. Part 409 is amended as follows: Section 409.5 is revised to read as follows:

§ 409.5 General description of benefits.

Hospital insurance (Part A of Medicare) helps pay for inpatient hospital services and posthospital SNF care. It also pays for home health services and hospice care. There are limitations on the number of days of care that Medicare can pay for and there are deductible and coinsurance amounts for which the beneficiary is responsible. For each type of service, certain conditions must be met as specified in the pertinent sections of this subpart and in Part 418 of this chapter regarding hospice care. Plus special conditions for inpatient hospital services furnished by a qualified U.S., Canadian, or Mexican hospital are set forth in Part 405, Subpart A of this chapter.

H. A new Part 418 is added as set forth below:

PART 418—HOSPICE CARE

Subpart A—General Provisions and Definitions

Sec.
418.1 Statutory basis.
418.2 Scope of part.

Source: Reprinted from *Federal Register,* Vol. 48, No. 243, pp. 56026–56036, December 16, 1983.

418.3 Definitions.

Subpart B—Eligibility, Election and Duration of Benefits

418.20 Eligibility requirements.
418.22 Certification of terminal illness.
418.24 Election of hospice care.
418.26 Elements of the election statement.
418.28 Revoking the election of hospice care.
418.30 Change of the designated hospice.
418.32 Duration of hospice coverage under Medicare.

Subpart C—Conditions of Participation

418.50 Condition of participation—General provisions.

Administration

418.52 Condition of participation—Governing body.
418.54 Condition of participation—Medical director.
418.56 Condition of participation—Professional management.
418.58 Condition of participation—Plan of care.
418.60 Condition of participation—Continuation of care.
418.62 Condition of participation—Informed consent.
418.64 Condition of participation—Inservice training.
418.66 Condition of participation—Quality assurance.
418.68 Condition of participation—Interdisciplinary group.
418.70 Condition of participation—Volunteers.
418.72 Condition of participation—Licensure.
418.74 Condition of participation—Central clinical records.

Core Services

418.80 Condition of participation—Core services.
418.82 Condition of participation—Nursing services.
418.84 Condition of participation—Medical social services.
418.86 Condition of participation—Physician services.
418.88 Condition of participation—Counseling services.

Other Services

418.90 Condition of participation—Other services.
418.92 Condition of participation—Physical therapy, occupational therapy, and speech-language pathology.
418.94 Condition of participation—Home health aide and homemaker services.
418.96 Condition of participation—Medical supplies.
418.98 Condition of participation—Short-term inpatient care.

Freestanding Hospice With Inpatient Unit

418.100 Condition of participation for freestanding hospices providing inpatient care directly.

Subpart D—Covered Services

418.200 Requirements for coverage.
418.202 Covered services.
418.204 Special coverage requirements.

Subpart E—Reimbursement Methods

418.301 Reimbursement for hospice care.
418.302 Payment procedures for hospice care.
418.304 Payment for physician services.
418.306 Determination of payment rates.
418.308 Limitation on the amount of hospice payment.
418.309 Hospice cap amount.
418.310 Reporting and recordkeeping requirements.
418.311 Administrative appeals.

Subpart F—Coinsurance

418.400 Individual liability for coinsurance for hospice care.
418.402 Individual liability for services that are not considered hospice care.
418.405 Reduction of Medicare reimbursement for individual coinsurance liability.
Authority: Secs. 1102, 1811-1814, 1861-1866, and 1871 of the Social Security Act (42 U.S.C. 1395c-1395f, 1395x-1395cc and 1395hh).

Subpart A—General Provision and Definitions

§ 418.1 Statutory basis.

This part implements Secs. 1861(dd) of the Social Security Act. Section 1861(dd) specifies services covered as hospice care and the conditions that a hospice program must meet in order to participate in the Medicare program. The following sections of the Act are also pertinent:
 (a) Sections 1812(a)(4) and (d) of the Act specify eligibility requirements for the individual and the benefit periods.
 (b) Section 1813(a)(4) of the Act specifies coinsurance amounts.
 (c) Sections 1814(a)(8) and 1814(i) of the Act contained conditions and limitations on coverage of and reimbursement for hospice care.
 (d) Sections 1862(a)(1), (6) and (9) of the Act established limits on hospice coverage.

§ 418.2 Scope of part.

Subpart A of this part sets forth the statutory basis and Scope and defines terms used in this part. Subpart B specifies the eligibility requirements and the benefit periods. Subpart C specifies conditions of participation for hospices. Subpart D describes the covered services and specifies the limits on services covered as hospice care. Subpart E specifies the reimbursement methods and procedures. Subpart F specifies coinsurance amounts applicable to hospice care.

§ 418.3 Definitions.

For purposes of this part—

"Attending physician" means a physician who—

(a) Is a doctor of medicine or osteopathy, and

(b) Is identified by the individual, at the time he or she elects to receive hospice care, as having the most significant role in the determination and delivery of that individual's medical care.

"Bereavement counseling" means counseling services provided to that individual's family after that individual's death.

"Cap period" means the twelve-month period ending October 31 used in the application of the cap on the overall hospice reimbursement specified in § 418.309.

"Carrier" means an organization that has a contract with HCFA to administer Medicare's supplementary medical insurance program.

"Election period" means one of three periods for which an individual may elect to receive Medicare coverage of hospice care. The periods consist of two 90-day periods and one 30-day period.

"Employee" means employee (defined by section 210(j) of the Act) of the hospice or, if the hospice is a subdivision of an agency or organization, an employee of the agency or organization who is appropriately trained and assigned to the hospice unit. "Employee" also refers to a volunteer under the jurisdiction of the hospice.

"Freestanding Hospice" means a hospice that is not part of any other type of participating provider.

"Hospice" means a public agency or private organization or subdivision of either of these that—

(a) Is primarily engaged in providing care to terminally ill individuals; and

(b) Meets the conditions specified in §§418.50-418.98 and has a valid provider agreement and if it is a freestanding hospice that provides inpatient care directly, meets the condition in §418.100.

"Intermediary" means an organization that has a contract with the Secretary to administer the benefits covered by Medicare's hospital insurance program, including the benefits covered under this part.

"Physician" means physician as defined in §405.232a of this chapter.

"Representative" means a person who is, because of the individual's mental or physical incapacity, authorized in accordance with State law to execute or revoke an election for hospice care or terminate medical care on behalf of the terminally ill individual.

"Social worker" means a person who has at least a bachelor's degree from a school accredited or approved by the Council on Social Work Education.

"Terminally ill" means that the individual has a medical prognosis that his or her life expectancy is 6 months or less.

Subpart B—Eligibility, Election and Duration of Benefits

§ 418.20 Eligibility requirements

In order to be eligible to elect hospice care under Medicare, an individual must be—

(a) Entitled to Part A of Medicare; and
(b) Certified as being terminally ill in accordance with § 418.22.

418.22 Certification of terminal illness.

(a) *Obtaining certification.* The hospice must obtain the certification that an individual is terminally ill in accordance with the following procedures:

(1) For the first 90-day period of hospice coverage, the hospice obtains, no later than two calendar days after hospice care is initiated, written certification statements signed by—

(i) The medical director of the hospice or the physician member of the hospice interdisciplinary group; and

(ii) The individual's attending physician if the individual has an attending physician.

(2) For the subsequent 90-day or 30-day period, the hospice obtains, no later than two calendar days after the beginning of that period, a written certification statement prepared by the medical director of the hospice or the physician member of the hospice's interdisciplinary group.

(b) *Certification statement.* The certification must include—

(1) The statement that the individual's medical prognosis is that his or her life expectancy is six months or less; and

(2) The signature(s) of the physician(s) required to certify the terminal illness under paragraph (a) of this section.

(c) *Maintaining a record.* The hospice maintains the certification statements.

§ 418.24 Election of hospice care.

(a) *Election statement.* And if an individual who meets the eligibility requirements for hospice care elects to receive that care, he or she must file an election statement with a particular hospice. An election may also be filed by a representative as defined in § 418.3. The election statement must include the elements specified in § 418.26.

(b) *Sequence of election periods.* The two 90-day election periods must be used before the 30-day period.

(c) *Duration of election.* An election to receive hospice care will be considered to continue through the initial election period and through the subsequent election periods without a break in care as long as the individual—

(1) Remains in the care of a hospice; and

(2) Does not revoke the election under the provisions of § 418.28.

(d) *Effective date of election.*

(1) An individual or representative may designate any effective date for the election period that begins with the first day of hospice care or any subsequent day of hospice care.

(2) An individual or representative may not designate an effective date that is earlier than the date that the election is made.

(e) *Waiver of other benefits.* An individual waives all rights to Medicare payments for the duration of the election of hospice care for the following services:

(1) Hospice care provided by a hospice other than the hospice designated by the individual (unless provided under arrangements made by that designated hospice).

(2) Any Medicare services that are related to the treatment of the terminal condition for which hospice care was elected or a related condition or that are equivalent to hospice care except for services—

(i) Provided by that designated hospice;

(ii) Provided by another hospice under arrangements made by the designated hospice; and

(iii) Provided by the individual's attending physician if that physician is not an employee of the designated hospice or receiving compensation from the hospice for those services.

§ 418.26 Elements of the election statement.

The election statement must include the following:

(a) Identification of the particular hospice that will provide care to the individual.

(b) The individual's or representative's acknowledgement that he or she has been given a full understanding of the palliative rather than curative nature of hospice care, as it relates to the individual's terminal illness.

(c) Acknowledgement that certain Medicare services are waived by the election.

(d) The effective date of the election.

(e) The signature of the individual or representative.

§ 418.28 Revoking the election of hospice care.

(a) An individual or representative may revoke the individual's election of hospice care at any time during an election period.

(b) To revoke the election of hospice care, the individual or representative must file a statement with the hospice that includes the following information:

(1) A signed statement that the individual or representative revokes the individual's election for Medicare coverage of hospice care for the remainder of that election period.

(2) The date that the revocation is to be effective. (An individual or representative may not designate an effective date earlier than the date that the revocation is made.)

(c) An individual, upon revocation of the election of Medicare coverage of hospice care for a particular election period—

(1) Is no longer covered under Medicare for hospice care;

(2) Resumes Medicare coverage of the benefits waived under §418.24(e)(2); and

(3) May at any time elect to receive hospice coverage for any other hospice election periods that he or she is eligible to receive.

§ 418.30 Change of the designated hospice.

(a) An individual or representative may change, once in each election period, the designation of the particular hospice from which hospice care will be received.

(b) The change of the designated hospice is not a revocation of the election for the period in which it is made.

(c) To change the designation of hospice programs, the individual or representative must file, with the hospice from which care has been received and with the newly designated hospice, a statement that includes the following information:

(1) The name of the hospice from which the individual has received care and the name of the hospice from which he or she plans to receive care.

(2) The date that change is to be effective.

§ 418.32 Duration of hospice coverage under Medicare.

(a) *General rule.* Except as provided under paragraph (b) of this section, Medicare coverage of hospice care will end on September 30, 1986.

(b) *Exception.* Medicare coverage of hospice care will continue beyond September 30, 1986, for an individual who has an election in effect on that date. Medicare coverage of hospice care will continue for that individual until—

(1) The end of the election period in effect; and

(2) The end of any consecutive election period(s) that the individual would have been entitled to on September 30, 1986.

Subpart C—Conditions of Participation

§ 418.50 Condition of participation—General provisions.

(a) *Standard: Compliance.* A hospice must maintain compliance with the conditions in §§418.50-418.98. A freestanding hospice that provides inpatient services directly must also maintain compliance with the condition in §418.100.

(b) *Standard: Required services.* A hospice must be primarily engaged in providing the care and services described in §418.202, must provide bereavement counseling and must—

(1) Make nursing services, physician services, and drugs and biologicals routinely available on a 24-hour basis;

(2) Make all other covered services available on a 24-hour basis to the extent necessary to meet the needs of individuals for care that is reasonable and necessary for the palliation and management of terminal illness and related conditions; and

(3) Provide these services in a manner consistent with accepted standards of practice.

(c) *Standard: Disclosure of information.* The hospice must meet the disclosure of information requirements at §420.206 of this chapter.

Administration

§ 418.52 Condition of participation—Governing body.

A hospice must have a governing body that assumes full legal responsibility for determining, implementing and monitoring policies governing the hospice's total operation.

The governing body must designate an individual who is responsible for the day to day management of the hospice program.

The governing body must also ensure that all services provided are consistent with accepted standards of practice.

§ 418.54 Condition of participation—Medical director.

The medical director must be a hospice employee who is a doctor of medicine or osteopathy who assumes overall responsibility for the medical components of the hospice's patient care program.

§ 418.56 Condition of participation—Professional management.

Subject to the conditions of participation pertaining to services in §§ 418.80 and 418.90, a hospice may arrange for another individual or entity to furnish services to the hospice's patients. If services are provided under arrangement, the hospice must meet the following standards:

(a) *Standard: Continuity of care.* The hospice program assures that continuity of patient/family care in home outpatient, and inpatient settings.

(b) *Standard: Written agreement.* The hospice has a legally binding written agreement for the provision of arranged services. The agreement includes at least the following:

(1) Identification of the services to be provided.

(2) A stipulation that services may be provided only with the express authorization of the hospice.

(3) The manner in which the contracted services are coordinated, supervised, and evaluated by the hospice.

(4) The delineation of the role(s) of the hospice and the contractor in the admission process, patient/family assessment, and the interdisciplinary group care conferences.

(5) Requirements for documenting that services are furnished in accordance with the agreement.

(6) The qualifications of the personnel providing the services.

(c) *Standard: Professional management responsibility.* The hospice retains professional management responsibility for those services and ensures that they are furnished in a safe and effective manner by persons needing the qualifications of this part, and in accordance with the patient's plan of care and the other requirements of this part.

(d) *Standard: Financial responsibility.* The hospice retains responsibility for payment for services.

(e) *Standard: Inpatient care.* The hospice ensures that inpatient care is furnished only in a facility which meets the requirements in § 418.98 and its arrangement in any legally binding written agreement that meets the requirements of paragraph (b) and that also specifies, at a minimum—

(1) That the hospice furnishes to the inpatient provider a copy of the patient's plan of care and specifies the inpatient services to be furnished;

(2) That the inpatient provider has established policies consistent with those of the hospice and agrees to abide by the patient care protocols established by the hospice for its patients;

(3) That the medical record includes a record of all inpatient services and events and that a copy of the discharge summary and, if requested, a copy of the medical record are provided to the hospice;

(4) The party responsible for the implementation of the provisions of the agreement; and

(5) That the hospice retains responsibility for appropriate hospice care training of the personnel who provide the care under the agreement.

§ 418.58 Conditions of participation—Plan of care.

A written plan of care must be established and maintained for each individual admitted to a hospice program, and that care provided to an individual must be in accordance with the plan.

(a) *Standard: Establishment of plan.* The plan must be established by the attending physician, a medical director or physician designee and interdisciplinary group prior to providing care.

(b) *Standard: Review of plan.* The plan must be reviewed and updated, at intervals specified in the plan, by the attending physician, the medical director or physician designee and interdisciplinary group. These reviews must be documented.

(c) *Standard: Content of plan.* The plan must include assessment of the individual's needs and identification of the services including the management of discomfort and symptom relief. It must state in detail the scope and frequency of services needed to meet the patient's and family's needs.

§ 418.60 Condition of participation—Continuation of care.

A hospice may not discontinue or diminish care provided to a Medicare beneficiary because of the beneficiary's inability to pay for that care.

§ 418.62 Condition of participation—Informed consent.

A hospice must demonstrate respect for an individual's rights by ensuring that an informed consent form that specifies the type of care and services that may be provided as hospice care during the course of the illness has been obtained for every individual, either from the individual or representative as defined in § 418.3.

§ 418.64 Condition of participation—Inservice training.

A hospice must provide an ongoing program for the training of its employees.

§ 418.66 Condition of participation—Quality assurance.

A hospice must conduct an ongoing, comprehensive, integrated, self-assessment of the quality and appropriateness of care provided, including inpatient care, home care and care provided under arrangements. The findings are used by the hospice to correct identified problems and to revise hospice policies if necessary. Those responsible for the quality assurance program must—

(a) Implement and report on activities and mechanisms for monitoring the quality of patient care;

(b) Identify and resolve problems; and

(c) Make suggestions for improving patient care.

§ 418.68 Condition of participation—Interdisciplinary group.

The hospice must designate an interdisciplinary group or groups composed of individuals who provide or supervise the care and services offered by the hospice.

(a) *Standard: Composition of group.* The hospice must have an interdisciplinary group or groups that include at least the following individuals who are employees of the hospice:

(1) A doctor of medicine or osteopathy.

(2) A registered nurse.

(3) A social worker.

(4) A pastoral or other counselor.

(b) *Standard: Role of group.* The interdisciplinary group is responsible for—
(1) Participation in the establishment of the plan of care;
(2) Provision or supervision of hospice care and services;
(3) Periodic review and updating of the plan of care for each individual receiving hospice care; and
(4) Establishment of policies governing that day-to-day provision of hospice care and services.
(c) If a hospice has more than one interdisciplinary group, it must designate in advance the group it chooses to execute the functions described in paragraph (b)(4) of this section.
(d) *Standard: Coordinator.* The hospice must designate a registered nurse to coordinate the implementation of the plan of care for each patient.

§ 418.70 Condition of participation—Volunteers.

The hospice in accordance with the numerical standards, specified in paragraph (e) of this section, uses volunteers, and in defined roles, under the supervision of a designated hospice employee.
(a) *Standard: Training.* The hospice must provide appropriate orientation and training that is consistent with acceptable standards of hospice practice.
(b) *Standard: Role.* Volunteers must be used in administrative or direct patient care roles.
(c) *Standard: Recruiting and retaining.* The hospice must document active and ongoing efforts to recruit and retain volunteers.
(d) *Standard: Cost saving.* The hospice must document the cost savings achieved through the use of volunteers. Documentation must include—
(1) The identification of necessary positions which are occupied by volunteers;
(2) The work time spent by volunteers occupying those positions; and
(3) Estimates of the dollar costs which the hospice would have incurred if paid employees occupied the positions identified in paragraph (d)(1) for the amount of time specified in paragraph (d)(2).
(e) *Standard: Level of activity.* A hospice must document and maintain a volunteer staff sufficient to provide administrative or direct patient care in an amount that, at a minimum, equals 5 percent of the total patient care hours of all paid hospice employees and contract staff. The hospice must document a continuing level of volunteer activity. Expansion of care and services achieved through the use of volunteers, including the type of services and the time worked, must be recorded.
(f) *Standard: Availability of clergy.* The hospice must make reasonable efforts to arrange for visits of clergy and other members of religious organizations in the community to patients who request such visits and must advise patients of this opportunity.

§ 418.72 Condition of participation—Licensure.

The hospice and all hospice employees must be licensed in accordance with applicable Federal, State and local laws and regulations.
(a) *Standard: Licensure of program.* If State or local law provides for licensing of hospices, the hospice must be licensed.
(b) *Standard: Licensure of employees.* Employees who provide services must be licensed, certified or registered in accordance with applicable Federal or State laws.

§ 418.74 Condition of participation—Central clinical records.

In accordance with accepted principles of practice, the hospice must establish and maintain a clinical record for every individual receiving care and services. The record must be complete, promptly and accurately documented, readily accessible and systematically organized to facilitate retrieval.

(a) *Standard: Content.* Each clinical record is a comprehensive compilation of information. Entries are made for all services provided. Entries are made and signed by the person providing the services. The record includes all services whether furnished directly or under arrangements made by the hospice. Each individual's record contains—

(1) The initial and subsequent assessments;
(2) The plan of care;
(3) Identification date;
(4) Consent and authorization and election forms;
(5) Pertinent medical history; and
(6) Complete documentation of all services and events (including evaluations, treatments, progress notes, etc.).

(b) *Standard: Protection of information.* The hospice must safeguard the clinical record against loss, destruction and unauthorized use.

Core Services

§ 418.80 Condition of participation—Core services.

A hospice must ensure that substantially all the core services described in §§ 418.82-418.88 are routinely provided directly by hospice employees. A hospice may use contracted staff if necessary to supplement hospice employees in order to meet the needs of patients during periods of peak patient loads or under extraordinary circumstances. If contracting is used, the hospice must maintain professional, financial, and administrative responsibility for the services and must assure that the qualifications of staff and services provided meet the requirements specified in §§ 418.82-418.88.

§ 418.82 Conditions of participation—Nursing services.

The hospice must provide nursing care and services by or under the supervision of a registered nurse.

(a) Nursing services must be directed and staffed to assure that the nursing needs of patients are met.
(b) Patient care responsibilities of nursing personnel must be specified.
(c) Services must be provided in accordance with recognized standards of practice.

§ 418.84 Condition of participation—Medical social services.

Medical social services must be provided by a qualified social worker, under the direction of a physician.

§ 418.86 Conditions of participation—Physician services.

In addition to palliation and management of terminal illness and related conditions, physician employees of the hospice, including the physician member(s) of the interdisciplinary group, must also meet the general medical needs of the patients to the extent that these needs are not met by the attending physician.

§ 418.88 Condition of participation—Counseling services.

Counseling services must be available to both the individual and the family. Counseling includes bereavement counseling, providing after the patient's death as well as dietary, spiritual and any other counseling services for the individual and family provided while the individual is enrolled in the hospice.

(a) *Standard: Bereavement counseling.* There must be an organized program for the provision of bereavement services under the supervision of a qualified professional. The plan of care for these services should reflect family needs, as well as a clear delineation of services to be provided and the frequency of service delivery (up to one year following the death of the patient). A special coverage provision for bereavement counseling is specified § 418.204(c).

(b) *Standard: Dietary counseling.* Dietary counseling, when required, must be provided by a qualified individual.

(c) *Standard: Spiritual counseling.* Spiritual counseling must include notice to patients as to the availability of clergy as provided in § 418.70(f).

(d) *Standard: Additional counseling.* Counseling may be provided by other members of the interdisciplinary group as well as by other qualified professionals as determined by the hospice.

Other Services

§ 418.90 Condition of participation—Other services.

A hospice must ensure that the services described in §§ 418.92-418.98 are provided directly by hospice employees or under arrangements made by the hospice as specified in § 418.56.

§ 418.92 Condition of participation—Physical therapy, occupational therapy, and speech-language pathology.

Physical therapy services, occupational therapy services, and speech-language pathology services must be available, and when provided, offered in a manner consistent with accepted standards of practice.

§ 418.94 Condition of participation—Home health aide and homemaker services.

Home health aide and homemaker services must be available and adequate in frequency to meet the needs of the patients. A home health aide is a person who meets the training, attitude and skill requirements specified in § 405.1227 of this chapter.

(a) *Standard: Supervision.* A registered nurse must visit the home site at least every two weeks when aide services are being provided, and the visit must include an assessment of the aide services.

(b) *Standard: Duties.* Written instructions for patient care are prepared by a registered nurse. Duties include, but may not be limited to, the duties specified in § 405.1227(a) of this chapter.

§ 418.96 Condition of participation—Medical supplies.

Medical supplies and appliances including drugs and biologicals, must be provided as needed for the palliation and management of the terminal illness and related conditions.

(a) *Standard: Administration.* All drugs and biologicals must be administered in accordance with accepted standards of practice.

(b) *Standard: Controlled drugs in the patient's home.* The hospice must have a policy for the disposal of controlled drugs maintained in the patient's home when those drugs are no longer needed by the patient.

(c) *Standard: Administration of drugs and biologicals.* Drugs and biologicals are administered only by the following individuals:

(1) A licensed nurse or physician.

(2) An employee who has completed a State-approved training program in medication administration.

(3) Any other individual in accordance with applicable State and local laws. The persons and each drug and biological they are authorized to administer must be specified in the patient's plan of care.

§ 418.98 Condition of participation—Short term inpatient care.

Inpatient care must be available for pain control, symptom management and respite purposes, and

Must be provided in a participating Medicare or Medicaid facility.

(a) *Standard: Inpatient care for symptom control.* Inpatient care for pain control and symptom management must be provided in one of the following:

(1) A hospice that meets the condition of participation for providing inpatient care directly as specified in § 418.100.

(2) A hospital or an SNF that also meets the standards specified in § 418.100 (a) and (f) regarding 24-hour nursing service and patient areas.

(b) *Standard: Inpatient care for respite purposes.* Inpatient care for respite purposes must be provided by one of the following:

(1) A provider specified in paragraph (a) of this section.

(2) An ICF that also meets the standards specified in § 418.100 (a) and (f) regarding 24-hour nursing service and patient areas.

(c) *Standard: Inpatient care limitation.* Except as provided in paragraph (d) of this section, the total number of inpatient days used by Medicare beneficiaries who elected hospice coverage in any 12-month period preceding a certification survey in a particular hospice may not exceed 20 percent of the total number of hospice days for this group of beneficiaries.

(d) *Standard: Exemption from limitation.* Until October 1, 1986, any hospice that began operation before January 1, 1975 is not subject to the limitation specified in paragraph (c).

Freestanding Hospice With Inpatient Unit

§ 418.100 Condition of participation for freestanding hospices providing inpatient care directly.

A freestanding hospice that provides inpatient care directly must comply with all of the following standards.

(a) *Standard: Twenty-four-hour nursing service.*

(1) The facility provides 24-hour nursing services which are sufficient to meet total nursing needs and which are in accordance with the patient plan of care. Each patient receives treatments, medications, and diet as prescribed, and is kept comfortable, clean, well-groomed, and protected from accident, injury, and infection.

(2) Each shift must include a registered nurse who provides direct patient care:

(b) *Standard: Disaster preparedness.* The hospice has an acceptable written plan, periodically rehearsed with staff, with procedures to be followed in the event of an internal or external disaster and for the care of casualties (patients and personnel) arising from such disasters.

(c) *Standard: Health and safety laws.* The hospice must meet all Federal, State, and the local laws, regulations, and those pertaining to health and safety, such as provisions regulating—

(1) Construction, maintenance, and equipment for the hospice;

(2) Sanitation;

(3) Communicable and reportable diseases; and

(4) Post mortem procedures.

(d) *Standard: Fire protection.* Except as provided in paragraph (e) of this section, the hospice must meet the health-care occupancy provisions of the 1981 edition of the Life Safety Code of the National Fire Protection Association which is incorporated by reference.[1]

(e) *Standard: Fire protection waivers.*

(1) In consideration of a recommendation by the State survey agency, HCFA may waive specific provisions of the Life Safety Code required by paragraph (d) of this section, for as long as it considers appropriate, if—

(i) The waiver would not adversely affect the health and safety of the patient; and

(ii) Rigid application of specific provisions of the Code would result in unreasonable hardship for the hospice.

(2) Any facility of two or more stories that is not of fire resistive construction and is participating on the basis of a waiver of construction type or height, may not house blind, nonambulatory, or physically handicapped patients above the street-level floor unless the facility—

(j) Is one of the following construction types (as defined in the Life Safety Code)—

(A) Type II (1, 1, 1)—protected noncombustible;

(B) Fully sprinklered Type II (0, 0, 0)— noncombustible;

(C) Fully sprinklered Type III (2, 1, 1)—protected ordinary;

(D) Fully sprinklered Type V (1, 1, 1)— protected wood frame; or

(ii) Achieves a passing score on the Fire Safety Evaluation System (FSES).

(f) *Standard: Patient areas.*

(1) The hospice must design and equip areas for the comfort and privacy of each patient and family members.

---

[1]See footnote to §405.1022(b) of this chapter.

(2) The hospice must have—

(i) Physical space for private patient/family visiting;

(ii) Accommodations for family members to remain with the patient throughout the night;

(iii) Accommodations for family privacy after a patient's death;

(iv) Decor of which is homelike in design and function.

(3) Patients must be permitted to receive visitors at any hour, including small children.

(g) *Standard: Patient rooms and toilet facilities.* Patient rooms are designed and equipped for adequate nursing care and the comfort and privacy of patients.

(1) Each patient's room must—

(i) Be equipped with or conveniently located near toilet and bathing facilities;

(ii) Be at or above grade level;

(iii) Contain a suitable bed for patient and other appropriate furniture;

(iv) Have closet space that provides security and privacy for clothing and personal belongings;

(v) Contain no more than four beds;

(vi) Measure at least 100 square feet for a single patient room or 80 square feet for each patient for a multipatient room; and

(vii) Be equipped with a device for calling the staff member on duty.

(2) For an existing building, HCFA may waive the space and occupancy requirements of paragraphs (g)(1) (v) and (vi) of this section for as long as it is considered appropriate if it finds that—

(i) The requirements would result in unreasonable hardship on the hospice if strictly enforced; and

(ii) The waiver serves the particular needs of the patients and does not adversely affect their health and safety.

(h) *Standard: Bathroom facilities.* The hospice must—

(1) Provide an adequate supply of hot water at all times for patient use; and

(2) Have plumbing fixtures with control valves that automatically regulate the temperature of the hot water used by patients.

(i) *Standard: Linen.* The hospice has available at all times a quantity of linen essential for proper care and comfort of patients. Linens are handled, stored, processed, and transported in such a manner as to prevent the spread of infection.

(j) *Standard: Isolation areas.* The hospice must make provision for isolating patients with infectious diseases.

(k) *Standard: Meal service, menu planning, and supervision.* The hospice must—

(1) Serve at least three meals or their equivalent each day at regular times, with not more than 14 hours between a substantial evening meal and breakfast;

(2) Procure, store, prepare, distribute, and serve all food under sanitary conditions;

(3) Have staff member trained or experienced in food management or nutrition who is responsible for—

(i) Planning menus that meet the nutritional needs of each patient, following the orders of the patient's physician and, to the extent medically possible, the recommended dietary allowances of the Food and Nutrition Board of the National Research Council, National Academy of Sciences (Recommended Dietary Allowances [9th ed., 1981] is available from the Printing and Publications Office, National Academy of Sciences, Washington, D.C. 20418); and

(ii) Supervising the meal preparation and service to ensure that the menu plan is followed; and

(4) If the hospice has patients who require medically prescribed special diets, have the menus for those patients planned by a professionally qualified dietitian and supervise the preparation and serving of meals to ensure that the patient accepts the special diet.

(1) *Standard: Pharmaceutical hospice service.* The hospice provides appropriate methods and procedures for the dispensing and administering of drugs and biologicals. Whether drugs and biologicals are obtained from community or institutional pharmacists or stocked by the facility, the facility is responsible for drugs and biologicals for its patients, insofar as they are covered under the program and for ensuring that pharmaceutical services are provided in accordance with accepted professional principles and appropriate Federal, State, and local laws. (See § 405.1124(g), (h), and (i) of this chapter.)

(1) *Licensed pharmacist:* The hospice must—

(i) Employ a licensed pharmacist; or

(ii) Have a formal agreement with a licensed pharmacist to advise the hospice on ordering, storage, administration, disposal, and recordkeeping of drugs and biologicals.

(2) *Orders for medications.*

(i) A physician must order all medications for the patient.

(ii) If the medication order is verbal—

(A) The physician must give it only to a licensed nurse, pharmacist, or another physician; and

(B) The individual receiving the order, must record and sign it immediately and have the prescribing physician sign it in any manner consistent with good medical practice.

(3) *Administering medications.* Medications are administered only by one of the following individuals:

(i) A licensed nurse or physician.

(ii) An employee who has completed a State-approved training program in medication administration.

(iii) The patient if his or her attending physician has approved.

(4) *Control and accountability.* The pharmaceutical service has procedures for control and accountability of all drugs and biologicals throughout the facility. Drugs are dispensed in compliance with Federal and State laws. Records of receipt and disposition of all controlled drugs are maintained in sufficient detail to enable an accurate reconciliation. The pharmacist determines that drug records are in order and that an account of all controlled drugs is maintained and reconciled.

(5) *Labeling of drugs and biologicals.* The labeling of drugs and biologicals is based on currently accepted professional principles, and includes the appropriate accessory and cautionary instructions, as well as the expiration date when applicable.

(6) *Storage.* In accordance with State and Federal laws, all drugs and biologicals are stored in locked compartments under proper temperature controls and only authorized personnel have access to the keys. Separately locked compartments are provided for storage of controlled drugs listed in Schedule II of the Comprehensive Drug Abuse Prevention & Control Act of 1970 and other drugs subject to abuse, except under single unit package drug distribution systems in which the quantity stored is minimal and a missing dose can be readily detected. An emergency medication kit approved by the pharmaceutical services committee is kept readily available.

(7) *Drug disposal.* Controlled drugs no longer needed by the patient are disposed of in compliance with State requirements. In the absence of State requirements, the pharmacist and a registered nurse dispose of the drugs and prepare a record of the disposal.

Subpart D—Covered Services

§ 418.200 Requirements for coverage.

To be covered, hospice services must meet the following requirements. They must be reasonable and necessary for the palliation or management of the terminal illness as well as related conditions. The individual must elect hospice care in accordance with § 418.24 and a plan of care must be established as set forth in § 418.58 before services are provided. The services must be consistent with the plan of care. A certification that the individual is terminally ill must be completed as set forth in § 418.22.

§ 418.202 Covered services.

All services must be performed by appropriately qualified personnel, but it is the nature of the service, rather than the qualification of the person who provides it, that determines the coverage category of the service. The following services are covered hospice services:

(a) Nursing care provided by or under the supervision of a registered nurse.

(b) Medical social services provided by a social worker under the direction of a physician.

(c) Physicians' services performed by a physician as defined in § 405.232a of this chapter except that the services of the hospice medical director for the physician member of the interdisciplinary group must be performed by a doctor of medicine or osteopathy.

(d) Counseling services provided to the terminally ill individual and the family members or other persons caring for the individual at home. Counseling, including dietary counseling, may be provided both for the purpose of training the individual's family or other caregiver to provide care, and for the purpose of helping the individual and those caring for him or her to adjust to the individual's approaching death.

(e) Short-term inpatient care provided in a participating hospice inpatient unit, or a participating hospital or SNF, that additionally meets the standards in § 418.100 (a) and (f) regarding staffing inpatient areas. Services provided in an inpatient setting must conform to the written plan of care. Inpatient care may be required for procedures necessary for pain control or acute or chronic symptom management.

Inpatient care may also be furnished as a means of providing respite for the individual's family or other persons caring for the individual at home. Respite care must be furnished as specified in § 418.98(b). Payment for inpatient care will be made at the rate appropriate to the level of care as specified in § 418.302.

(f) Medical appliances and supplies, including drugs and biologicals. Only drugs as defined in section 1861(t) of the Act and which are used primarily for the relief of pain and symptom control related to the individual's terminal illness are covered. Appliances may include covered durable medical equipment as described in § 405.231(g) of this chapter as well as other self-help and personal comfort items related to the palliation or management of the patient's terminal illness. Equipment is provided by the hospice for use in the patient's home while he or she is under hospice care. Medical supplies include those that are part of the written plan of care.

(g) Home health aide services furnished by qualified aides as designated in § 418.94 and homemaker services. Home health aides may provide personal care services as described in § 405.127(d) of this chapter. Aides may also perform household services to maintain a safe and sanitary environment in areas of the home used by the patient, such as changing the bed or light cleaning and laundering essential to the comfort and cleanliness of the patient. Aide services must be provided under the general supervision of a registered nurse. Homemaker services may include assistance and personal care, maintenance of a safe and healthy environment and services to enable the individual to carry out the treatment plan.

(h) Physical therapy, occupational therapy and speech-language pathology services in addition to the services described in § 405.127(c) of this chapter provided for purposes of symptom control or to enable the patient to maintain activities of daily living and basic functional skills.

§ 418.204 Special coverage requirements.

(a) *Periods of crisis.* Nursing care may be covered on a continuous basis for as much as 24 hours a day during periods of crisis as necessary to maintain an individual at home. Either homemaker or home health aide services or both may be covered on a 24-hour continuous basis during periods of crisis but care during these periods must be predominantly nursing care. A period of crisis is a period in which the individual requires continuous care to achieve palliation or management of acute medical symptoms.

(b) *Respite care.* (1) Respite care is short-term inpatient care provided to the individual only when necessary to relieve the family members or other persons caring for the individual.

(2) Except as provided in paragraph (b)(3), respite care may be provided only on an occasional basis and may not be reimbursed for more than five consecutive days at a time.

(3) Until October 1, 1986, any hospice that began operation before January 1, 1975 is not subject to the limitation on the frequency and number of respite care days.

(c) *Bereavement counseling.* Bereavement counseling is a required hospice service but it is not reimbursable.

Subpart E— Reimbursement Methods

§ 418.301 Reimbursement for hospice care.

(a) Medicare payment for covered hospice care is made in accordance with the method set forth in § 418.302.

(b) Medicare reimbursement to a hospice in a cap period is limited to a cap amount specified in § 418.309.

§ 418.302 Payment procedures for hospice care.

(a) HCFA establishes payment amounts to reimburse specific categories of covered hospice care.

(b) Payment amounts are determined within each of the following categories:

(1) *Routine home care day.* A routine home care day is a day on which an individual who has elected to receive hospice care is at home and is not receiving continuous care as defined in paragraph (b)(2) of this section.

(2) *Continuous home care day.* A continuous home care day is a day on which an individual who has elected to receive hospice care is not in an inpatient facility and receives hospice care consisting predominantly of nursing care on a continuous basis at home. Home health aide or homemaker services or both may also be provided on a continuous basis. Continuous home care is only furnished during brief periods of crisis as described in § 418.204(a) and only as necessary to maintain the terminally ill patient at home.

(3) *Inpatient respite care day.* An inpatient respite care day is a day on which the individual who has elected hospice care receives care in an approved facility on a short-term basis for respite.

(4) *General inpatient care day.* A general inpatient care day is a day on which an individual who has elected hospice care receives general inpatient care and an inpatient facility for pain control or acute or chronic symptom management which cannot be managed in other settings.

(c) The payment amounts for the categories of hospice care are fixed payment rates that are calculated by HCFA in accordance with the procedures described in § 418.306. Payment rates are determined for the following categories:

(1) Routine home care.

(2) Continuous home care.

(3) Inpatient respite care.

(4) General inpatient care.

(d) The intermediary reimburses the hospice at the appropriate payment amount for each day for which an eligible Medicare beneficiary is under the hospice's care.

(e) The intermediary makes payment according to the following procedures:

(1) Payment is made to the hospice for each day during which the beneficiary is eligible and under the care of the hospice, regardless of the amount of services furnished on any given day.

(2) Payment is made for only one of the categories of hospice care described in § 418.302(b) for any particular day.

(3) On any day on which the beneficiary is not an inpatient, the hospice is paid the routine home care rate, unless the patient receives continuous care as defined in paragraph (b)(2) of this section for a period of at least 8 hours. In that case, a portion of the continuous care day rate is paid in accordance with paragraph (4) of this section.

(4) The hospice payment on a continuous care day varies depending on the number of hours of continuous services provided. The continuous home care rate is divided by 24 to yield an hourly rate. The number of hours of continuous care provided during a continuous home care day is then multiplied by the hourly rate to yield the continuous home care payment for that day. A minimum of 8 hours of care must be furnished on a particular day to qualify for the continuous home care rate.

(5) Subject to the limitations described in paragraph (f) of this section, on any day on which the beneficiary is an inpatient in an approved facility for inpatient care, the appropriate inpatient rate (general or respite) is paid for the date of admission and all subsequent inpatient days, except the day on which the patient is discharged. For the day of discharge, the appropriate home care rate is paid unless the patient dies as an inpatient. In the case where the beneficiary is discharged deceased, the inpatient rate (general or respite) is paid for the discharge day. Payment for inpatient respite care is subject to the requirement that it may not be provided consecutively for more than 5 days at a time. Payment for the sixth and any subsequent day of respite care is made at the routine home care rate.

(f) Payment for inpatient care is limited as follows:

(1) The total payment to the hospice for inpatient care (general or respite) is subject to a limitation that total inpatient care days for Medicare patients not exceed 20 percent of the total days for which these patients had elected hospice care.

(2) At the end of a cap period, the intermediary calculates a limitation on payment for inpatient care to ensure that Medicare payment is not made for days of inpatient care in excess of 20 percent of the total number of days of hospice care furnished to Medicare patients.

(3) If the number of days of inpatient care furnished to Medicare patients is equal to or less than 20 percent of the total days of hospice care to Medicare patients, no adjustment is necessary. Overall payments to a hospice are subject to the cap amount specified in § 418.309.

(4) If the number of days of inpatient care furnished to Medicare patients exceeds 20 percent of the total days of hospice care to Medicare patients, the total payment for inpatient care is determined in accordance with the procedures specified in paragraph (f)(5) of this section. That amount is compared to actual payments for inpatient care, and any excess reimbursement must be refunded by the hospice. Overall payments to the hospice are subject to the cap amount specified in § 418.309.

(5) If a hospice exceeds the number of inpatient care days described in paragraph (f)(4), the total payment for inpatient care is determined as follows:

(i) Calculate the ratio of the maximum number of allowable inpatient days to the actual number of inpatient care days furnished by the hospice to Medicare patients.

(ii) Multiply this ratio by the total reimbursement for inpatient care made by the intermediary.

(iii) Multiply the number of actual inpatient days in excess of the limitation by the routine home care rate.

(iv) Add the amounts calculated in paragraphs (f)(5)(ii) and (iii) of this section.

§ 418.304 Payments for physician services.

(a) The following services performed by hospice physicians are included in the rates described in § 418.302:

(1) General supervisory services of the medical director.

(2) Participation in the establishment of plans of care, supervision of care and services, periodic review and updating of plans of care, and establishment of governing policies by the physician member of the interdisciplinary group.

(b) For services not described in paragraph (a) of this section, a specified Medicare contractor pays the hospice an amount equivalent to 100 percent of the physician's reasonable charge for those physician services furnished by hospice employees or under arrangements with the hospice. Reimbursement for these physician services is included in the amount subject to the hospice payment limits described in § 418.309. Services furnished voluntarily by physicians are not reimbursable.

(c) Services of the patient's attending physician, if he or she is not an employee of the hospice or providing services under arrangements with the hospice, are not considered hospice services and are not included in the amount subject to the hospice payment limit described in § 418.309. These services are paid by the carrier under the procedures in Subparts D or E, Part 405 of this chapter.

§ 418.306 Determination of the payment rates.

(a) HCFA calculates payment rates for each of the categories of hospice care described in § 418.302(c).

(b) Each rate is equal to a prospectively determined amount which HCFA estimates equals the costs incurred by hospice generally and efficiently providing that type of hospice care to Medicare beneficiaries.

(c) The rates are adjusted by the intermediary to reflect local differences in wages.

(d) HCFA will publish as a notice in the Federal Register any proposal to change payment rates or the methodology for determining those rates.

§ 418.308 Limitation on the amount of hospice payments.

(a) Except as specified in paragraph (b) of this section, the total Medicare payment to a hospice for care furnished during a cap period is limited by the hospice cap amount specified in § 418.309.

(b) Until October 1, 1986, payment to a hospice that began operation before January 1, 1975 is not limited by the amount of the hospice cap specified in § 418.309.

(c) The intermediary notifies the hospice of the determination of program reimbursement at the end of the cap year in accordance with procedures similar to those described in 42 CFR 405.1803.

(d) Payments made to a hospice during cap period that exceed the cap amount are overpayments and must be refunded.

§ 418.309 Hospice cap amount.

The hospice cap amount is calculated using the following procedures:

(a) The cap amount is $6,500 per year and is adjusted for inflation or deflation for cap years that end after October 1, 1984, by using the percentage change in the medical care expenditures category of the Consumer Price Index (CPI) for urban consumers that is published by the Bureau of Labor Statistics. This adjustment is made using the change in the CPI from March 1984 to the fifth month of the cap year. The cap year runs from November 1 of each year until October 31 of the following year.

(b) Each hospice's cap amount is calculated by the intermediary by multiplying the adjusted cap amount determined in paragraph (a) of this section by the number of Medicare beneficiaries who elected to receive hospice care from that hospice during the cap period. For purposes of this calculation, the number of Medicare beneficiaries includes—

(1) Those Medicare beneficiaries who have not previously been included in the calculation of any hospice cap and who have filed an election to receive hospice care, in accordance with § 418.24, from the hospice during the period beginning on Sept. 28 (35 days before the beginning of the cap period) and ending on Sept. 27 (35 days before the end of the cap period).

(2) In the case in which a beneficiary has elected to receive care from more than one hospice, each hospice includes in its number of Medicare beneficiaries only that fraction which represents the portion of a patient's total stay in all hospices that was spent in that hospice. (The hospice can obtain this information by contacting the intermediary.)

§ 418.310 Reporting and recordkeeping requirements.

Hospices must provide reports and keep records as the Secretary determines necessary to administer the program.

§ 418.311 Administrative appeals.

A hospice that believes its payments have not been properly determined in accordance with these regulations may request a review from the intermediary or the Provider Reimbursement Review Board (PRRB) if the amount in controversy is at least $1,000 or

$100,0000, respectively. In such a case, the procedure in 42 CFR Part 405, Subpart R, will be followed to the extent that it is applicable. The PRRB, subject to review by the Secretary under § 405.1874 of this chapter, shall have the authority to determine the issues raised. The methods and standards for the calculation of the payment rates by HCFA are not subject to appeal.

Subpart F—Coinsurance

§ 418.400 Individual liability for coinsurance for hospice care.

An individual who has filed an election for hospice care in accordance with § 418.24 is liable for the following coinsurance payments. Hospices may charge individuals the applicable coinsurance amounts.

(a) *Drugs and biologicals.* An individual is liable for a coinsurance payment for each palliative drug and biological prescription furnished by the hospice while the individual is not an inpatient. The amount of coinsurance for each prescription approximates 5 percent of the cost of the drug or biological to the hospice determined in accordance with the drug copayment schedule established by the hospice, except that the amount of coinsurance for each prescription may not exceed $5. The cost of the drug or biological may not exceed what a prudent buyer would pay in similar circumstances. The drug copayment schedule must be reviewed for reasonableness and approved by the intermediary before it is used.

(b) *Respite care.* The amount of coinsurance for each respite care day is equal to 5 percent of the payment made by HCFA for a respite care day.

(2) The amount of the individual's coinsurance liability for respite care during a hospice coinsurance period may not exceed the inpatient hospital deductible applicable for the year in which the hospice coinsurance period began.

(3) The individual hospice coinsurance period—

(i) Begins on the first day an election filed in accordance with § 418.24 is in effect for the beneficiary; and

(ii) Ends with the close of the first period of 14 consecutive days on each of which an election is not in effect for the beneficiary.

§ 418.402 Individual liability for services that are not considered hospice care.

Medicare payment to the hospice discharges an individual's liability for payment for all services, other than the hospice coinsurance amounts described in § 418.400, that are considered covered hospice care (as described in § 418.202). The individual is liable for the Medicare deductibles and coinsurance payments and for the difference between the reasonable and actual charge on unassigned claims or other covered services that are not considered hospice care. Examples of services not considered hospice care include: services furnished before or after a hospice election period: services of the individual's attending physician, if the attending physician is not an employee of or working under an arrangement with the hospice; or Medicare services received for the treatment of an illness or injury not related to the individual's terminal condition.

§ 418.405 Reduction of Medicare reimbursement by individual coinsurance liability.

The Medicare payment rates established by HCFA in accordance with § 418.306 are not reduced when the individual is liable for coinsurance payments. Instead, when determining the payment rates, HCFA offsets the estimated cost of services by an estimate of average coinsurance amounts hospices collect.

PART 420—PROGRAM INTEGRITY

The authority citation for Part 420 reads as follows:
Authority: Secs. 1102, 1128, 1862(d), 1862(e), 1866(b)(2)(D), (E), and (F), 1871, 1902(a)(39), and 1903(i)(2) of the Social Security Act (42 U.S.C. 1302, 1320a-7, 1395y(d), 1395y(e), 1395cc(b)(2)(D), (E), and (F), 1395hh, 1396a(a)(39), and 1396b(i)(2)).

I. Part 420 is amended as follows:

1. In subpart A, § 420.2 is amended by revising the definition of "Provider" to read as follows:

Subpart A—General Provisions

* * * *

§ 420.2 Definitions.

* * * *

"Provider" means a hospital, a skilled nursing facility, a comprehensive outpatient rehabilitation facility, a home health agency, or a hospice that has in effect an agreement to participate in Medicare, or a clinic, a rehabilitation agency, or a public health agency that has a similar agreement, but only to furnish outpatient physical therapy or speech pathology services.

* * * *

2. In Subpart D, § 420.301, the introductory language is reprinted and the definition of "Provider" is revised to read as follows:

Subpart D—Access to Books, Documents, and Records of Subcontractors

* * * *

§ 420.301 Definitions.

For purposes of this subpart—

* * * *

"Provider" means a hospital, skilled nursing facility, home health agency, comprehensive outpatient rehabilitation facility, a hospice, or a related organization (as defined in § 407.427 of this chapter) of any of these providers.

* * * *

PART 421—INTERMEDIARIES AND CARRIERS

J. Part 421 is amended as follows:

1. The Table of Contents is amended by revising the title of § 421.117 to read as follows:

* * * *

Sec.

421.117—Designation of intermediaries for freestanding home health agencies and hospices.

* * * *

Authority: Secs. 1102, 1815, 1816, 1842, 1861(u), 1871, 1874 and 1875 of the Social Security Act (42 U.S.C. 1302, 1395g, 1395h, 1395u, 1395x(u), 1395hh, 1395kk, and 1395(l), and 42 U.S.C. 1395-1.

2. Section 421.3 is amended by revising the definitions of "Intermediary" and "Provider" to read as follows:

§ 421.3 Definitions.

* * * *

"*Intermediary*" means an organization that has entered into an agreement with the Administrator to perform designated functions in the administration of the Medicare program.

For purposes of designating intermediaries and freestanding home health agencies and hospices under § 421.117 as well as for applying the performance criteria in § 421.120 and the statistical standards in § 421.122 and any adverse action resulting from such application, the term intermediary also means a Blue Cross Plan which has entered into a subcontract approved by the Administrator with the Blue Cross Association to perform intermediary functions.

"*Provider*" means a hospital, skilled nursing facility (SNF), home health agency (HHA), hospice, comprehensive outpatient rehabilitation facility, or a provider of outpatient physical therapy or speech pathology services under the Medicare program.

* * * *

3. Section 421.103 is revised to read as follows:

§ 421.103 Options available to providers.

Except for hospices (which are covered under § 421.117), a provider may elect to receive payment for covered services furnished to Medicare beneficiaries:

(a) Directly from the Administrator, or

(b) Through an intermediary, when both the Administrator and the intermediary consent.

4. Section 421.104 is amended by revising paragraph (a)(1) to read as follows:

§ 421.104 Nominations for intermediary.

(a) *Nomination by groups or associations of providers.*

(1) An association of providers, except for hospices, may nominate an organization or agency to serve as intermediary for its members.

* * * *

5. Section 421.106 is amended by revising the introductory material in paragraph (a) to read as follows:

§ 421.106 Change to another intermediary or to direct payment.

(a) Any provider may request a change of intermediary, or except for a hospice, that it be billed directly by the Administrator, by—

* * * *

6. Section 421.117 is amended by revising the title and paragraph (a), and by adding a new paragraph (c) to read as follows:

§ 421.117 Designation of intermediaries for freestanding home health agencies and for hospices.

(a) This section is based on section 1816(e)(4) of the Social Security Act, which requires the Secretary to designate regional intermediaries for freestanding home health agencies (HHAs) and on section 1816(e)(5) of the Social Security Act, which requires the Secretary to designate intermediaries for hospices.

* * * *

(c) Except for certain hospice physician services, which generally are reimbursed by carriers, hospices receive payment for covered services furnished to Medicare beneficiaries in accordance with the following:

(1) Freestanding hospices receive payment through an intermediary designated by HCFA.

(2) Except as described in paragraph (c)(3), hospices that are subdivisions of other Medicare providers receive payment through the same intermediary that serves their parent provider.

(3) A hospice whose parent provider is served by HCFA receives payment through an intermediary designated by HCFA.

7. Section 421.128 is amended by revising paragraph (f) to read as follows:

§ 421.128 Intermediary's opportunity for a hearing and right to judicial review.

* * * *

(f) Exception. An intermediary adversely affected by the designation of an intermediary under § 421.117 of this subpart is not entitled to a hearing or judicial review concerning adverse effects caused by the designation of an intermediary.

PART 489—PROVIDER AGREEMENTS UNDER MEDICARE

The authority citation for Part 489 reads as follows:

Authority: Secs. 1102, 1814(a), 1861, 1864, 1866, and 1871 of the Social Security Act (42 U.S.C. 1302, 1395f(a), 1395x, 1395aa, 1395cc, and 1395hh).

K. Part 489 is amended as follows:

1. Section 489.2 is amended by adding a new paragraph (b)(6) to read as follows:

§ 489.2 Scope of part.

* * * *

(b) The following providers are subject to the provisions of this part:

* * * *

(6) Hospices.

2. Section 489.55 is amended by revising paragraph (b) to read as follows:

§ 409.55 Exceptions to effective date of termination.

* * * *

(b) In a case of home health services furnished under a plan of treatment or hospice care furnished under a plan of care established before the effective date, payment may be made for services furnished through the end of the calendar year in which termination is effective.

(Catalog of Federal Domestic Assistance Program No. 13773, Medicare Hospital Insurance)
Dated: October 31, 1983.
Administrator, Health Care Financing Administration.
Approved: Nov. 4, 1983.
Margaret M. Heckler,
Secretary
(FR Doc. 83-33331 Piled 12-13-83; 11:19am)
BILLING CODE 4120-03-M

PART VII

DEPARTMENT OF HEALTH AND HUMAN SERVICES

Health Care Financing Administration

42 CFR Parts 400, 405, 408, 409, 418, 420, 41, and 489

Medicare Program; Hospice Care and Prospective Payment for Medicare Inpatient Hospital Services; Correction; Final Rule

Medicare Program; Schedule of Target Rate Percentages for Limits on the Rate of Hospital Cost Increases and Updating Factors for Transition Prospective Payment Rates (Second Quarter FY 84); Correction; Notice

DEPARTMENT OF HEALTH AND HUMAN SERVICES

Health Care Financing Administration

42 CFR Parts 400, 405, 408, 409, 418, 420, 421, and 489

(BERC-242-CN/263-CN)

Medicare Program; Hospice Care and Prospective Payment for Medicare Inpatient Hospital Services; Correction

AGENCY: Health Care Financing Administration (HCFA), HHS.
ACTION: Correction to final rules.
SUMMARY: This document corrects errors that appeared in the final rule on hospice care published on December 16, 1983 (48 FR 56008) and the final rule on the prospective payment system for inpatient hospital services published on January 3, 1984 (49 FR 234). The former rule implemented section 122 of Pub. L. 97-248 providing coverage for hospice care and responded to comments received on a proposed rule published August 22, 1983 (48 FR 38146). The latter final rule amended, in response to public comments received, the interim final rule published on September 1, 1983 (48 FR 39752). In certain instances, we have made nonsubstantive changes in the prospective payment regulations text for purposes of clarification.
EFFECTIVE DATE: January 3, 1984.
FOR FURTHER INFORMATION CONTACT: William Rush, 301-594-9777.
SUPPLEMENTARY INFORMATION: In FR Doc. 83-33331, (the Hospice Care final regulations published December 16, 1983) beginning on page 56008, make the following corrections:

1. On page 56019, in the second column, in the 41st line, "$3.24" should read "$2.91."
2. On page 56032, in the second column, in the last sentence of § 418.100 (l)(6), remove "approved by the pharmaceutical services committee."

In FR Doc. 83-34405 (the Prospective Payment final regulations published January 3, 1984), beginning on page 234, make the following corrections:

Source: Reprinted from *Federal Register,* Vol. 49, No. 107, pp. 23010–23014, June 1, 1984.

1. On page 236, in the second column, in the first paragraph of the last full paragraph, "§ 405.471(c)(4)(ii)(E)(3)(i)" should read "§ 405.471(c)(4)(ii)(D)(3)(i)."

2. Also on page 236, in the third column, in the 11th line from the bottom, "§ 405.471(c)(4)(ii)(D)(4)," should read "§ 405.471(c)(4)(ii)(C)(4)," and the 10th line from the bottom, the phrase beginning with "which" and ending with "plan," should be removed.

3. On page 241, and the first column, in the 16th line from the top, within the parentheses, "§ 405.471(c)(4)(i)(G)" should read "§ 405.471(c)(3)(i)(G) in the interim final rule."

4. Also on page 241, in the second column, in the 15th line from the top, the second "of" should read "or."

5. On page 242, in the first column, in the third line from the top, "(c)(4)(ii)(C)" should read "(c)(4)(ii)(B)."

6. On page 245, in the first column, in the 38th line from the top, "quality" should read "qualify."

7. On page 248, in the first column, in the 12th line from the top, change "four" to "three."

8. On page 249, and the first column, in the second line of the second full paragraph, ".0515" should read ".5010."

9. Also on page 249, in the third column, in the first paragraph of item C, the cross reference should read "§ 405.470(b)(3)."

10. On page 251, in the third column, in the second line from the bottom, "(c)" should be capitalized.

11. One page 252, in the first column, in the first and fourth lines from the top, "For all" should read "for *all*."

12. Also on page 252, in the third column, following the first full paragraph and before the second paragraph beginning with " *Comment,*" add the following new paragraph:

"For the interested reader, the revised national standardized amounts for FY 84 have been calculated to be $2,825.58 as the urban average ($2,196.63 for about labor share and $628.95 for the nonlabor share) and $2,254.16 as the rural average ($1,839.39 for the labor share and $414.77 for the nonlabor share). As stated in the preamble to the interim final rule, these amounts are only estimates that, for comparison purposes, have been computed in the same manner as the regional amounts contained in Table 1, section VII of the addendum."

13. On page 253, in the second column, under item four, in the third sentence of the first response paragraph, add "area" between "rural" and "within"; and in the fourth sentence, "on" should read "one."

14. Also on page 253, in the third column, in the second through fifth lines from the top, remove "status of those hospitals which have been reclassified by paying at the appropriate standardized amounts for their revised," and in the last sentence of the first full paragraph, "other" should read "earlier."

15. On page 254, in the first column, in the first sentence of the last paragraph, insert "is" following "98-21."

16. On page 258, in the table in the center of the page, insert "S" before the following figures in the second line: 2.000.500, 1.913.88, and 500. Also, in the same table, in the last column to the right, "1.0450" should read "1.0450."

17. On page 259, in the first column, in the formula in the middle of the page, remove "Outlier adjustment X," and beginning in the 12th line from the bottom, remove the bullet point and "The intermediary reduces the case-mix adjusted based year costs to take into account outlier payments."

18. Also on page 259, in the second column, in the second line from the top, "D.3" should read "C.2."

19. On page 262, in the third column, in the ninth line from the top, "$35.000" should read "$35,000."

20. On page 267, in the third column, in the 11th line from the top, insert "should" between "hospital" and "be," and in the 15th line from the top, "if" should read "it."

21. On page 268, in the first column, beginning on the 14th line from the top, remove the entire parenthetical statement.

22. On page 271, in the first column, in the 16th line from the top, insert "regional" between "the" and "Federal," and beginning on the 17th line from the top, remove the phrase "of payment to SCHs."

23. On page 283, in the first column, in the fourth line, delete "the," and insert "covered" before the word "stays."

24. On page 293, in the first column, in the title of item D, "Physical" should read "Physician."

25. On page 295, in the first column, in the first response paragraph, in the eighth line, insert the following phrase between the words "the" and "hospitals": "statutory requirements concerning *extensive billing* and that immediate compliance would *threaten the stability of patient care*. We are optimistic that".

26. On page 300, in the first column, in the third line from the top, "§ 405.463(C)(5)(iii)" should read § 405.463(c)(5)(iii)," and beginning with the 22nd line from the top, revise the paragraph beginning with "Distinguish" and ending with "appealed," to read as follows:

"—Clarifying when, and to what extent, estimates of the based year costs by fiscal intermediaries are subject to administrative and judicial review."

27. Also on page 300, in the second column, beginning with the second indented point in section F, revise the paragraph beginning with "Section" and ending with "services," to read as follows:

"Section 405.476(b)(3)(ii)(B) was changed to permit a rural hospital, located between 25 and 50 miles from other like hospitals, to be classified as an SCH if it meets one of three stated criteria. We added a provision, regarding the 25 percent utilization criteria, that permits, if data on general resident utilization are not available, use of the Medicare beneficiary utilization percentage in the service area. Additionally, we will permit classification as an SCH if the hospital has less than 50 beds and the PSRO or intermediary certifies that the hospital would have met the above criteria (that is, 25 percent utilization) except that beneficiaries or residents were forced to seek care outside the service area due to the unavailability of needed specialty services."

28. On page 307, in the first column, in the second line of the second full paragraph, insert "come" between "not" and "into."

29. Also on page 307, in the second column, in the sixth sentence of the first paragraph under item H.1., delete "With this exception," and begin the sentence with "Over."

30. On page 309, in the first column, in the third sentence of the first full paragraph, insert "1886" after "section."

31. On page 310, in the third column, in the fifth line, "$151" should read "$197."

32. On page 311, in the first column, the second full paragraph should be revised to read as follows: "In addition, as noted above in section IV.C.1. of this preamble, we removed paragraph (b)(5) of § 405.474, which concerned outlier adjustments in the determination of the hospital-specific rate. This change is effective with cost reporting periods beginning on or after October 1, 1983."

33. On page 312, in the second column, in the amendatory language and authority citation for subpart D of Part 405, in the ninth line from the bottom, "reads," should be changed to "is revised to read," and in the fifth line from the bottom, "1395(a)" should read "1395l(a)."

34. On page 313, in the third column, in the amendatory language for § 405.463, the second line under item 7 should read "(h)(1) (i), (ii), and (iii) or revised to read as."

35. On page 314, in § 405.463, in the first column, following paragraph (h)(1)(ii) and preceding the five stars, add paragraph (h)(1)(iii) to read as follows:

(iii) HCFA may adjust the amount of operating costs, under paragraph (c)(1) of this section, to take into account factors such as a change in the inpatient hospital services that a hospital provides, that are customarily provided directly by similar hospitals, or the manipulation of discharges to increase reimbursement. A change in the inpatient hospital services provided could result from changes that include, but are not limited to, opening or closing a special care unit or changing the arrangement under which such services may be furnished, such as leasing a department.

36. On page 315, in the second column, in the eighth line from the top in § 405.471(c)(3)(viii), insert a comma after "houses" and remove "and" before the word "recovery"; and in the ninth line from the top, insert "with" between " and" and "self-help."

37. On page 316, in the second column, in § 405.471(c)(4)(iii), "distant" should read "distinct."

38. On page 317, in the first column, in the last line under item 10, "and (e)(3)" should read "(e)(3), (e)(4), and (e)(5)."

39. On page 317, in the first column, the introductory language of paragraph (b)(1) under § 405.472 should be revised to read as follows:

(b) *Charge to beneficiaries.*

(1) *Permitted charges*—stay covered. A hospital receiving payment under the prospective payment system for a covered hospital stay (that is, a state that includes at least one covered day) may charge the Medicare beneficiary or other person only for the following items and services furnished during that stay—

40. Also on page 317, in the first column, paragraph (b)(1)(ii) under § 405.472 should be revised to read as follows:

(ii) Noncovered items and services, furnished at any time during a covered stay, unless they are excluded from coverage only on the basis of the following:

(A) The exclusion of custodial care under § 405.310(g) (see paragraph (b)(1)(iii) of this section for when charges may be made for custodial care);

(B) By exclusion of medically unnecessary items and services under § 405.310(k) (see paragraphs (b)(1) (iii) and (iv) of this section for when charges may be made for medically unnecessary items and services);

(C) The exclusion under § 405.310(m) of nonphysician services furnished to hospital inpatients by other than the hospital or a provider or supplier under arrangements made by the hospital;

(D) The exclusion of items and services furnished when the patient is not entitled to Medicare Part A benefit under Subpart A of Part 408 of this chapter (see paragraph (b)(1)(v) of this section for when charges may be made for items and services furnished when the patient is not entitled to benefit); or

(E) By exclusion of items and services furnished after Medicare Part A benefit are exhausted under § 409.61 of this chapter (see paragraph (b)(1)(v) of this section for when charges may be made for items and services furnished after benefits are exhausted);

41. On page 317, in the second column, in § 405.472(b)(1)(iii)(A), beginning with the 12th line from the top, revise the parenthetical statement to read "(The phrase "inpatient hospital care" includes cases where a beneficiary needs a SNF level of care, but, under Medicare criteria, a SNF-level bed is not available.

This also means that a hospital may find that a patient awaiting SNF placement no longer requires inpatient hospital care because either a SNF-level bed has become available or the patient no longer requires SNF-level care.)."

42. On page 318, in the second column, following paragraph (e)(3), and paragraphs (e)(4) and (e)(5) to read as follows:

(4) Any person furnishing services described in paragraph (e)(1) of this section who is dissatisfied with a determination made by the Office of the Inspector General under paragraph (e)(3) is entitled to reasonable notice and opportunity for a hearing thereon to the same extent as is provided in section 205(b) of the Act and to judicial review of the final decision after such hearing as is provided in section 205(g).

(5) The Office of the Inspector General will promptly notify each State agency which administers or supervises the administration of a State plan approved under title XIX of the Act of any determination made under the provisions of paragraph (e)(3) of this section.

* * * *

43. Also on page 318, in the second column, item 11 is revised to read as follows:

11. Section 405.474 is amended by revising paragraphs (b) and (c)(1) to read as follows:

44. Also, beginning on page 318, in § 405.474, in the second column following the title to § 405.474 and five stars, and ending on page 319, in the first column before paragraph (c), for purposes of general verification and to clarify that a provider's rights to appeal become available upon receipt of its notice of amount of program reimbursement following the close of its cost reporting period, paragraphs (b)(1) through (b)(8) should be added or revised to read as follows:

* * * *

(b) *Determining the hospital-specific rate*—(1) *Base-year costs.* (i) For each hospital, the intermediary will estimate the hospital's Medicare Part A allowable inpatient operating costs, as described in § 405.470(b)(3), for the 12-month or longer cost reporting period ending on or after September 30, 1982 and before September 30, 1983.

(ii) If the hospital's last cost reporting period ending before September 30, 1983 is for less than 12 months, the base period will be the hospital's most recent 12-month or longer cost reporting period ending before such short-period report, with an appropriate adjustment for inflation. (See paragraph (c) of this section for rules applicable to new hospitals.)

(2) *Modifications to base year costs.*

(i) Prior to determining the hospital-specific rate, the intermediary will adjust the hospital's estimated base year inpatient operating costs, as necessary, to eliminate nursing differential costs (as described in § 405.430), direct medical education costs (as described in § 405.421), capital-related costs (as described in § 405.414), and kidney acquisition costs incurred by hospitals approved as renal transplantation centers (as described in § 405.476(h)). Kidney acquisition costs in the base year will be determined by multiplying the hospital's average kidney acquisition cost per kidney times the number of kidney transplants covered by Medicare Part A during the base period. Malpractice insurance costs will be included in the inpatient operating costs, as described in § 405.452. Also, higher costs that were incurred for purposes of increasing base year costs, or either one-time non-recurring higher costs or revenue offsets that have the effect of distorting base year costs as an appropriate basis for computing the hospital-specific rate or higher costs that result from changes in hospital accounting principles initiated in the base year, will be excluded from base year costs for purposes of this section.

(ii) Prior to that date it becomes subject to the prospective payment system, a hospital may request the intermediary to further adjust its estimated base period costs to take into account—

(A) Services paid for under Medicare Part B during the hospital's base year that will be paid for under prospective payment. The base year costs may be increased to include estimated payments for certain services previously billed as physicians' services before the effective date of § 405.550(b), and estimated payments for nonphysicians' services that were not furnished either directly or under arrangements before October 1, 1983 (the effective date of § 405.310(m)), but may include the costs of anesthetists' services for which a physician employer continues to bill under § 405.553(b)(4).

(B) The payment of FICA taxes during cost reporting periods subject to the prospective payment system, if the hospital had not paid such taxes for all its employees during its base period and will be required to participate effective January 1, 1984.

(iii) If a hospital requests its base period costs to be adjusted under paragraph (b)(2)(ii) of this section, it must timely provide the intermediary with sufficient documentation to justify the adjustment and adequate data to compute the adjusted cost. The intermediary will decide whether to use part or all of the data based on audit, survey and other information available.

(3) *Limitations on modifying calculations.*

(i) The intermediary will use the best data available at the time in estimating each hospital's base year costs and the modifications to those costs authorized by paragraph (b)(2) of this section. The intermediary's estimate of base year costs and modifications thereto is final and may not be changed after the first day of the first cost reporting period beginning on or after October 1, 1983, except as follows:

(A) A hospital that becomes subject to the prospective payment system beginning on or after October 1, 1983 and before November 16, 1983, may request its intermediary up to November 15, 1983, to reestimate its base period costs to take into account inadvertent omissions in its previous submissions to the intermediary related to changes made by the prospective payment legislation for purposes of estimating the base period costs. The intermediary may also initiate changes to the estimation for any reason prior to the date the hospital becomes subject to prospective payment, and before November 16, 1983, for corrections to take into account inadvertent omissions in the hospital's previous submissions related to changes made by the prospective payment legislation for purposes of estimating the base period costs. Such omissions pertain to adjustments to exclude capital-related costs and the direct medical education costs of approved educational activities and to adjustments specified in paragraph (b)(2)(ii) of this section. The intermediary must notify the provider of any change to the hospital-specific amount as a result of the provider's request within 30 days of receipt of the additional data. Any change to base period costs made persuant to the above exception will be made effective retroactively, beginning with the first day of the affected hospital's fiscal year.

(B) To correct mathematical errors of calculations. The hospital must report such errors of calculations to the intermediary within 90 days of that intermediary's notification to the hospital of the hospital's payment rates. The intermediary may also identify such errors and initiate their correction during this period. The intermediary will either make an appropriate adjustment or notify the hospital that no adjustment is warranted within 30 days of receipt of the hospital's report of an error. Corrections of errors of calculation will be effective with the first day of the hospital's first cost reporting period subject to the prospective payment system.

(C) To take into account a successful appeal of the provider's base period notice of amount of program reimbursement under Subpart R of this part. If a hospital successfully contests a disallowance of costs incurred in its base year, the intermediary will recalculate the hospital's base year costs, incorporating the additional costs recognized as allowable as a result of the appeal. Adjustments to base period costs to take into account such previously disallowed costs will be effective with the first day of the hospital's first cost reporting period beginning on or after the date of the appeal decision. The hospital's revised base period costs will not be used to recalculate the hospital-specific portion as determined for fiscal years beginning before the date of the appeal decision.

(D) To take into account a successful appeal relating to modifications to base year costs that were made pursuant to paragraph (b)(2) of this section. If a hospital successfully contests a modification to base year costs, the intermediary will recalculate the hospital's base year costs to reflect the modification determined appropriate as a result of the appeal. Such adjustments will be effective retroactively to the time of the intermediary's initial estimation of base year costs.

(E) To exclude costs that were unlawfully claimed as determined as a result of criminal conviction, imposition of a civil judgment under the False Claims Act (31 U.S.C. 3729-3731), or a proceeding for exclusion from the Medicare program. In addition to adjusting base year costs, HCFA will recover both the excess costs reimbursed for the base period and the additional amounts due to the inappropriate increase of the hospital-specific portion of the hospital's transition payment rates. The amount to be recovered will be computed based on the final resolution of the amount of the inappropriate base-year costs.

(iii) An intermediary's estimation of a hospital's base year costs, and modifications thereto, made for purposes of determining the hospital-specific rate, is subject to administrative and judicial review (available to a hospital upon receipt of its notice of amount of program reimbursement following the close of its cost reporting period (see §§ 405.1803 and 1807)) only with respect to whether the intermediary followed the provisions of this paragraph (b). In any administrative or judicial review of whether the intermediary used the best data available at the time, as required by paragraph (b)(3)(i) of this section, an intermediary's estimation will be revised only on this review only if the estimation was unreasonable and clearly erroneous in light of the data available at the time the estimation was made. Specifically excluded from administrative or judicial review are any issues based on data, information, or arguments not presented to the intermediary at that time of the estimation.

(4) *Costs on a per discharge basis.* The intermediary will determine the hospital's estimated adjusted base year operating cost per discharge by dividing the total adjusted operating costs by the number of discharges in the base period.

(5) *Case-mix adjustment.* The intermediary will divide the adjusted base year costs by the hospital's 1981 case-mix index. If the hospital's case-mix index is statistically unreliable (as determined by HCFA), the hospital's base year costs will be divided by the lower of:

(i) The hospital's estimated case-mix index; or

(ii) The average case-mix index for the appropriate classifications of all hospitals subject to cost limits, established under § 405.460 for cost reporting periods beginning on or after October 1, 1982 and before October 1, 1983.

(6) *Updating base year costs.*

(i) *For Federal fiscal year 1984.* The case-mix adjusted base year cost per discharge will be updated by the applicable updating factor (that is, the target rate percentage determined under § 405.463(c)(3), as adjusted for budget neutrality.

(ii) *For Federal fiscal year 1985.* The amount determined under paragraph (b)(6)(i) of this section will be updated by the applicable updating factor, as adjusted for budget neutrality.

(iii) *For Federal fiscal year 1986.* The amount determined under paragraph (b)(6)(ii) of this section will be updated by the applicable updating factor, that is, the target rate percentage determined under § 405.463(c)(3).

(7) *Budget neutrality.*

(i) *Federal fiscal year 1984.* For cost reporting periods beginning on or after October 1, 1983 and before October 1, 1984, HCFA will adjust the target rate percentage used under paragraph (b)(6) of this section by a factor actuarially estimated to ensure that the estimated amount of aggregate Medicare payments made based on the hospital-specific portion of the transition payment rates are neither greater nor less than 75 percent of the payment amounts that would have been payable for the inpatient operating costs for those same hospitals for fiscal year 1984 under the law in effect before April 20, 1983.

(ii) *Federal fiscal year 1985.* For cost reporting periods beginning on or after October 1, 1984 and before October 1, 1985, HCFA will adjust the target rate percentage used under paragraph (b)(6) of this section by a factor actuarially estimated to ensure that the estimated amount of aggregate Medicare payment made based on the hospital-specific portion of the transition payment rates are neither greater nor less than 50 percent of the payment amounts that would have been payable for the inpatient operating costs for those same hospitals for fiscal year 1985 under the Social Security Act as in effect on April 19, 1983.

(8) *DRG adjustment.* The applicable hospital-specific cost per discharge will be multiplied by about appropriate DRG weighting factor to determine the hospital-specific base payment amount (target amount) for a particular covered discharge.

45. On page 319, in the second column, the amendatory language in the item 12 should read as follows:

12. Section 405.475 is amended by revising the title of paragraph (c), and paragraphs (c)(1), (c)(2), (c)(3), (c)(4), (d)(3), and (d)(6) to read as follows:

46. Also on page 319, in the second column in the introductory language of § 405.475(c)(2), following the word "approve", add "to the extent required by HCFA—".

47. Also on page 319, in § 405.475(c)(3), in the second column, following the table, remove the five stars, and insert paragraph (c)(4) to read as follows:

(4) Any days in a covered stay identified as noncovered will reduce the number of days reimbursed at the day outlier rate but not to exceed the number of days which occur after the day outlier threshold.

48. Also on page 319, in the second column in § 405.475(d)(3), beginning with the eighth line of text from the bottom, revised paragraph (d)(3) to read as follows:

* * * *

(d) *Payment for extraordinarily high cost cases (cost outliers).*

(1) * * *

(3) The hospital must request review of all services by a medical review entity. Payment cannot be made for non-approved services. The entity, at the direction of HCFA, using the medical records and itemized charges, must determine whether:

(i) The admission was medically necessary and appropriate.

(ii) Services were medically necessary and delivered in the most appropriate setting.

(iii) Services were actually rendered, ordered by the physician, and not duplicatively billed, and

(iv) The diagnostic and procedural coding are correct.

* * * *

49. Also on page 319, in the third column, in § 405.475(d)(6), in the second line from the top, "(3)" should read "(4)".

50. On page 320, in § 405.476(g)(2), in the second column, in the eighth line from the top, "(c)(6)" should read "(c)(5)".

51. Also on page 320, in the second column in § 405.477(d)(2)(v)(B), insert "and" after "hospital".

52. Also on page 320, in the second column in § 405.477(e)(3), in the fourth line from the bottom, "Part P" should read " Part B", and "Part B payment to outside suppliers." should be italicized.

53. Also on page 320, in the third column in § 405.1042(c)(2)(i), in the fifth line from the bottom, "§ 405.575(a)(1)" should read "§ 405.475(a)(1)".

54. On page 321, in the first column, in § 405.1627(a)(1)(ii), "§ 405.470" should read "§ 405.475".

55. Also on page 321, in the second column, in the title of § 405.1627(e)(1) after "the" insert "prospective".

56. On page 322, in the first and second columns, items (1) and (2), under that definition of "Intermediary determination" in § 405.1801(a), are revised to read as follows:

§ 405.1801 Introduction.

(a) *Definitions.* * * * *

"Intermediary determination" means the following:

(1) With respect to a provider of services that has filed a cost report under §§ 405.406 and 405.453(f), the term means a determination of the amount of total reimbursement to the provider, pursuant to § 405.1803 following the close of the provider's cost reporting period, for items and services furnished to beneficiaries for which reimbursement may be made on a reasonable cost basis under Medicare for the period covered by the cost report.

(2) With respect to a hospital that receives payments for inpatient hospital services under the prospective payment system (§§ 405.470-405.477), the term means a determination of the total amount of payment to the hospital, pursuant to § 405.1803 following the close of the hospital's cost reporting period, under that system for the period covered by the determination.

* * * *

57. On page 325, in the second column, in the first line of item C.1., "(c)" should be capitalized.

58. On page 326, in the second column, in the second line from the top, insert "(" before "20.85%)".

59. On page 328, in the second column, in the 25th line from the top, remove "(Transmittal 291)".

60. Also on page 328, in the third column, in the fourth line from the bottom, insert "1 plus" between "to" and "the".

61. On page 329, in the first column, in the fourth line from the bottom, insert "meet the criteria in § 405.474(c)(ii) or that" between "that" and "have".

62. On page 333, in the second column, in the second paragraph under item F., change the reference "section III." To read "section IV.C.".

(Secs. 1102, 1814(b), 1815, 1833(a), 1861(v), 1862(a), 1871, 1876, 1881, 1883, 1886, and 1887 of the Social Security Act, as amended (42 U.S.C. 1302, 1395f(b), 1395g, 1395l(a), 1395x(v), 1395y(a), 1395hh, 1395mm, 1395rr, 1395tt, 1395ww, and 1395xx))

(Catalog of Federal Domestic Assistance Programs No. 13.773. Medicare—Hospital Insurance: No. 13.774, Medicare—Supplementary Medical Insurance.)

Dated: May 4, 1984.

Carolyne K. Davis,

Administrator, Health Care Financing Administration.

Approved: May 29, 1984.

Margaret M. Heckler,

Secretary.

(FR Doc. 84-14889 Filed 5-31-84; 11:32 am)

BILLING CODE 4120-03-M

DEPARTMENT OF HEALTH AND HUMAN SERVICES

Health Care Financing Administration

42 CFR Part 418

(BERC-30-F)

Medicare Program; Hospice " Core" Service; Nursing

AGENCY: Health Care Financing Administration (HCFA), HHS.
ACTION: Final rule.
SUMMARY: These final regulations permit certain hospices located in areas that are not urbanized to receive from HCFA a waiver of the requirement to provide nursing services directly. The regulations implement section 2343 of the Deficit Reduction Act of 1984 (Pub. L. 98-369).
DATE: These final regulations are effective on April 10, 1987.
FOR FURTHER INFORMATION CONTACT: Thomas Hoyer, (301) 594-9446.
SUPPLEMENTARY INFORMATION:

I. Background

A. Introduction of hospice care

Hospice care is an approach to treatment that recognizes that the impending death of an individual warrants a change in focus from curative care to palliative care. The goal of hospice care is to help terminally ill individuals continue life with minimal disruption in normal activities while remaining primarily in the home environment. A hospice uses an interdisciplinary approach to deliver medical, social, psychological, emotional, and spiritual services through the use of a broad spectrum of professional and other care-givers with the goal of making the individual as physically and emotionally comfortable as possible.

The hospice experience in the United States has placed emphasis on home care. It offers physician services, specialized nursing services, and other forms of care in the home in order to enable the terminally ill individual to remain at home in the company of family and friends as long as possible. Inpatient hospice settings have been used when the individual's pain and symptoms must be closely monitored in order to be controlled, when medical intervention is required to control pain or palliate symptoms, or when the family needs a rest from the stress involved in caring for the individual (respite care).

B. Legislative History

Section 122 of the Tax Equity and Fiscal Responsibility Act (TEFRA) of 1982 (Pub. L. 97-248, enacted on September 3,1982) enacted section 1861(dd) of the Social Security Act (Act) to expand the scope of Medicare benefits by all authorizing coverage for hospice care for terminally ill beneficiaries with a life expectancy of six months or less. Section 1861(dd)(2)(A)(ii)(I) of the Act specifies that a hospice must routinely provide directly substantially all of the following "core services": nursing care, medical social services, physicians' services and counseling services. The remaining "non-core services" may be provided either directly by the hospice or under arrangements with others, in which case the hospice must maintain professional management responsibility for all such services

---

Source: Reprinted from *Federal Register,* Vol. 52, No. 47, pp. 7412–7416, March 11, 1987.

furnished to an individual, regardless of the location of or type of facility in which such services are furnished.

On July 18, 1984 section 2343 of the Deficit Reduction Act of 1984 (DRA), Pub. L. 98-369, amended section 1861(dd) of the Act by adding a new paragraph (5), to permit the Secretary to waive, for certain hospices, the requirement that a hospice routinely provide directly substantially all nursing services. Section 1861(dd)(5)(A) of the Act specifies that to obtain a waiver a hospice must be located in an area that is not an urbanized area (as defined by the Bureau of the Census), must have been in operation on or before January 1, 1983, and must demonstrate a good faith effort (as determined by the Secretary) to hire a sufficient number of nurses to provide nursing care directly. Section 1861(dd)(5)(B) of the Act specifies that if a waiver is requested by an organization that meets the statutory requirements, and if it is submitted in the format and contains the information required by the Secretary, the waiver will be deemed granted unless the request is denied by the Secretary within 60 days after the request is received by the Secretary. Further, that paragraph states that the granting of a waiver will not preclude the favorable consideration of a subsequent waiver request should such a request be necessary.

Section 2343 of DRA specifies that the Secretary must study the necessity and appropriateness of the "core services" requirement and submit the findings to Congress prior to January 1, 1986. (This date corresponds to the date that the Secretary must submit a report concerning the hospice program's reimbursement method and benefit structure.) The study must include not only an analysis of Medicare-approved hospices but also a review of non-Medicare hospices. Although this report has not yet been submitted because of the difficulty of obtaining the necessary information, research reports are being compiled and we expect that we will submit the report in early 1987.

C. Current Regulations

We published a final rule on December 16, 1983 (48 FR 56008) to implement the hospice program under Medicare (42 CFR Part 418). The final rule defines a hospice as a public agency or private organization or subdivision of either of these that is primarily engaged in providing care to terminally ill individuals, meets the conditions specified in the regulations and has a valid provider agreement.

The December 16, 1983 final rule requires that a hospice provide nursing care and services by or under the supervision of a registered nurse (42 CFR 418.82) and that the services routinely be provided directly by hospice employees (42 CFR 418.80). Under these regulations, a hospice may use contracted staff to meet the "core service" needs of its patients, but only when necessary to supplement hospice employees during periods of the patient loads or under extraordinary circumstances.

On March 3, 1986, we published in the Federal Register a proposed regulation (51 FR 7292) to implement section 2343 of Pub. L. 98-369 concerning waiving the requirement for certain hospices routinely to provide directly substantially all nursing services.

II. Provisions of the Proposed Regulations

As evidenced by the amendment to this statute, Congress was concerned that the original law and current regulations may have placed an unreasonable burden on hospices located in rural areas by requiring them to provide nursing care services directly. Rural hospices have reported problems in hiring enough nurses to provide hospice care, and they have also questioned the cost-effectiveness of directly employing nurses in rural areas where hospice utilization is relatively low.

We proposed on March 3, 1986 to implement the statutory provision that permits the Secretary to waive the requirement that an agency or organization must routinely provide directly substantially all of the nursing "core services" for certain agencies or organizations with respect to all or part of the nursing care. Hospices that are located in non-urbanized areas (as identified by the Bureau of the Census) and were operational on or before January 1, 1983, may be given a waiver of the requirement that nursing services be provided directly if they can demonstrate that they made a good-faith effort to hire nurses. This waiver may involve nursing services throughout the hospice's service area or, for a hospice which functions in a large non-urban area where availability of nurses differs from one location to another, may be granted only for a part of the hospice's service area. The proposed rule would have made the waivers granted under this authority effective for one year.

The statute permits the Secretary to set forth the form and information required in order to determine whether to grant the waiver. The statute and our criteria require that the hospice demonstrate an effort at recruitment which failed.

As required by the statute, we proposed to make determinations as to urbanized and non-urbanized areas based on current Census Bureau designations. For a hospice which operates in several areas, the location of the hospice would be considered the location of its central office. We proposed to determine whether a hospice was operational on or before January 1, 1983 based on:

1. Proof that the organization was established to provide hospice services on or before January 1, 1983 (for example, newspaper advertisements, dated correspondence on hospice letterhead, dated invoices, articles of incorporation, governing body minutes);

2. Evidence that hospice-type services were actually furnished to patients on or before January 1, 1983 (for example, dated copies of medical records, nursing notes, pharmaceutical orders); and

3. Evidence that the hospice care was a discrete activity rather than an aspect of another type of provider's patient care program on or before January 1, 1983 (that is, evidence of a distinct program in an existing provider or articles of incorporation that show it to be a discrete and separate organization).

We proposed to adopt these criteria because we recognize that most of these hospices would not have been able to meet the full range of requirements set forth in section 1861(dd)(2) of the Act, the statutory definition of "hospice program," since the definition did not exist until the enactment of the provision. Nonetheless, it is clear that the basic statutory concept of a hospice is of a discrete activity providing hospice care and that, therefore, these waivers should be restricted to such hospices.

We proposed to make determinations of good faith efforts to hire nurses based on the following:

1. Proof of recruitment efforts through advertisements in professional journals or local newspapers;

2. Copies of job descriptions for nurse employees;

3. Evidence that salary and benefits are competitive for the area (for example, evidence of salary and benefits offers in connection with recruitment advertisements); and

4. Any other contributing activities (for example, recruiting efforts at health fairs).

We were especially interested in comments concerning the appropriateness of the above criteria and any suggestions for other items and we specifically requested comments/suggestions in the proposed rule.

We proposed that a hospice would submit a request for waiver of the nursing core services requirement directly to HCFA. We proposed to respond to all requests within 60 days; however, any waiver request would, under the law, be deemed to be granted unless it is denied within 60 days after it is received. The granting of a waiver would not preclude the favorable consideration of a subsequent waiver request should such a request be necessary.

III. Analysis of and Responses to Public Comments

We received 11 pieces of correspondence from national hospice, hospital, and nurses' organizations; State agencies; and health care providers commenting on the proposed rule. In drafting this final regulation, we considered all comments. The comments and our responses to these comments are discussed below.

A. General Comment

Comment: One commenter requested that we state in regulations that the granting of a waiver would not preclude favorable consideration of a subsequent waiver request should such a request be necessary.

Response: We do not believe it necessary to state in regulations that the granting of a waiver would not preclude favorable consideration of a subsequent waiver request should such a request be necessary. The regulation states the conditions for granting waivers and the length of time for each waiver.

Core Services Waiver Requirements

Comment: Five organizations commented on the statement that the location of a hospice that operates in several areas is considered to be the location of its central office (§ 418.83(a)). These commenters believe that this definition unnecessarily restricts eligibility for the waiver and that waivers should be allowed for hospices or parts of hospices that perform most of their services in rural locations. One of these commenters also suggested that HCFA should not permit hospices that were in operation by January 1, 1983, to expand, relocate, or otherwise begin operating in rural areas so that they may qualify for a waiver. The commenter noted that any manipulation that results in a hospice being allowed to operate on a Statewide basis through the granting of a waiver would negate the intent of the statutory core services requirement.

Response: In developing the proposed regulations, we were careful to avoid either exceeding or narrowing the statutory scope of the waiver. When we approve a hospice for Medicare participation, the approved unit is essentially the central office of the provider, although the provider is responsible for services furnished throughout its service area. In this respect, we are following a policy we have used for many years in determining the location of a provider for purposes of determining its Medicare payment status (for example, which wage index to apply to its services). Although we recognize that a hospice may provide services in areas that are somewhat distant from its central office, we do not believe that these areas should be considered separate entities for purposes of allowing this waiver. To do so would divide the hospice into unmanageable parts for purposes of Medicare participation and for purposes of its own personnel management. The creation of this waiver authority was not for the purpose of allowing hospices to expand their service areas beyond their capacity to care directly for patients. A hospice service area should be such that a hospice can directly manage the care of its patients. The waiver was enacted to permit hospices to exist in rural areas where a shortage of nurses would otherwise preclude it from meeting the core services requirement and we are providing for partial waivers not to permit undue expansion in rural areas but to assure that a waiver is granted only to the extent that it is needed to permit the hospice to function. Admittedly, there exists the possibility that an urban hospice may experience a similar problem; however, section 1861(dd)(5)(A) of the Act permits waivers only for hospices located in non-urban areas. Because we consider the location of a hospice to be the location of its central office, we will not approve waivers for hospices whose central offices are located in urban areas. An additional concern is that allowing waivers in parts of an urban hospice's non-urban service area could encourage expansion to even more remote areas where the hospice's control of the services provided would be questionable and monitoring would be infeasible. We agree with the commenter who suggested that we not allow waivers for hospices that relocate or otherwise begin operating in rural areas so as to qualify for a waiver. We will address this issue in guidelines.

Comment: Three organizations commented on the requirement that an applicant submit evidence that the hospice was a discrete activity rather than an aspect of another type of provider's care program on or before January 1, 1983 (§ 418.83(a)(2)). One commenter believes that this requirement appears to narrow eligibility unnecessarily and the other two commenters requested clarification of the type of evidence that would be expected. The commenters suggested several examples of possible evidence, including articles of incorporation, records indicating that hospice-type care was provided by a separate department, and accounting records that indicate a separate cost center.

Response: This requirement is designed to implement the statutory requirement that the agency or organization was in operation on or before January 1, 1983. We recognize that home health agencies, hospitals, and other providers may have provided special care to terminal patients for many years. Because the Medicare hospice benefit is relatively new, we did not specify any particular model for the hospice-type care provided on or before January 1, 1983, but we believe that it is essential to establish that the hospice care provided was a distinct and organized activity rather than general care provided to terminal patients who were part of the provider's general patient population. All of the examples of evidence that the commenters suggested and any other evidence that indicates that the hospice activity was distinct from the provider's general care may be submitted. We do not believe that it is appropriate to limit the range of materials that may be submitted by listing acceptable evidence and regulations.

Comment: Five organizations commented on the requirement concerning evidence that would demonstrate a good faith effort to hire nurses (§ 418.83(a)(3)). One group suggested that we require that recruitment efforts be undertaken within the six months preceding the date that a waiver is requested. Another organization suggested that we provide more specificity concerning competitiveness of the salary and benefits offered. Two organizations suggested that we list items of evidence as examples rather than requiring that all items be submitted. One organization requested that we require a copy of an advertisement in a local newspaper and not allow an advertisement in a professional journal to be substituted for this evidence because the newspaper advertisement is much more likely to come to the attention of a nurse in the locale. This commenter also suggested that evidence of a recruitment plan include contacting nurses in other health care settings such as visiting nurse association's, public health departments and hospitals.

Response: While we believe these suggestions are useful, we do not believe it appropriate to include them in regulations. We plan to incorporate many of them into our manual instructions when we publish interim instructions for the Hospice Manual (HCFA Pub. 21), the State Operations Manual (HCFA Pub. 7), the Part A Intermediary Manual (HCFA Pub. 13), and the Regional Office Manual (HCFA Pub. 23). These instructions will provide details relating to submission of waiver requests. With respect to the local newspaper advertisement for recruiting nurses, we have accepted that comment and changed the regulations accordingly (§ 418.83(a)(3)(i)).

Comment: Three groups commented that the proposed one-year duration of a waiver (§ 418.83(c)) is too short in view of the substantial recruitment efforts and documentation required to obtain a waiver. One commenter also noted that the employment market for nurses is unlikely to change in the course of one year. All three commenters suggested a three-year waiver period.

Response: We believe the commenters raised a valid concern. Accordingly, although we have retained a one-year waiver period, we have added a provision permitting a maximum of two one-year extensions (§ 418.83(d)). Under this provision, if a hospice wishes to receive a one-year extension, the hospice must submit a certification to HCFA, prior to the expiration of the waiver period, that the employment market for nurses has not changed significantly since the time the initial waiver was granted. In the event that new Census Bureau designations are made during the course of a waiver period (including any extension), and the hospice is no longer located in a non-urbanized area, the initial waiver will remain in effect until the end of the approved period.

C. Contracting for Nurses

Comment: Three commenters believe that a waiver should be granted if a hospice can establish that it would be more cost-effective to contract for nurses than to hire them or if a small hospice is too poor to hire nurses. One commenter suggested that contracting be allowed so as to avoid staff burnout.

Response: We have no statutory authority to provide waivers for hospices on any basis other than those described in section 1861(dd)(5)(A) of the Act, which relates only to the inability of hospices in certain locations to recruit nurses.

IV. Summary of Changes in the Final Regulations

As stated in our discussion of the comments and responses, we have made some changes to the approach we had proposed in the regulations published on March 3, 1986. With the exception of the changes identified below, the final regulations reflect the proposals made in the March 3, 1996 proposed rule.

A. Evidence of Recruitment Efforts to Hire Nurses

We have revised § 418.83(a)(3)(i) to require a hospice to demonstrate recruitment efforts to hire nurses by providing us with copies of local newspaper advertisements. We eliminated the option of advertisements in professional journals as proof of recruitment efforts. We have also included "contracts with nurses at other providers in the area" as an example of recruiting activities in §418.83(a)(3)(iv).

B. Duration of Waiver Period

We have extended the duration of the waiver period to three years. In the event that new Census Bureau designations are made during the course of a waiver period, and the hospice is no longer located in a non-urbanized area, the waiver would remain in effect until the end of the approved three-year period.

C. Census Bureau Designations

We inadvertently included in § 418.83(a)(1) of the proposed regulations a reference to the "1980" Bureau of the Census designations for determining non-urbanized areas. The statute does not require the use of the 1980 designations. In the final regulations, we have deleted the reference to "1980". The Bureau of the Census updates its designations every ten years and we will use the most current designations available when the waiver application is received.

V. Impact Analysis

Executive Order 12291 (E.O. 12291) requires us to prepare and publish regulatory impact analysis for regulations that are likely to meet criteria for a "major rule". A major rule is one that will result in: (1) an annual effect on the economy of $100 million or more; (2) a major increase in costs or prices for consumers, individual industries, Federal, State, or local government agencies, or any geographic regions; or (3) significant adverse effects on competition, employment, investment, productivity, innovation or the ability of the United State-based enterprises to compete with foreign-based enterprises in domestic or export markets.

In addition, consistent with the Regulatory Flexibility Act (RFA) (5 U.S.C. 601-612), we prepare and published a regulatory flexibility analysis for regulations unless the Secretary certifies that the regulations will not have a significant impact on a substantial number of small entities. For purposes of the RFA, we consider all for-profit and most not-for-profit providers to be small entities.

As noted elsewhere in this preamble, section 2343 of Pub. L. 98-369, seeks to correct an unreasonable burden that may have been created by the original law and the current regulations. Specifically, Congress concluded that rural hospices were encountering problems in hiring enough nurses to provide hospice care directly. This final rule permits certain rural hospices to request a waiver that will provide them administrative flexibility in securing nursing services. Since the main test for obtaining a waiver is the demonstrated inability to recruit nurse employees, we expect that virtually no existing hospices (which have already been approved for Medicare participation) will be applying successfully for a waiver. Rather, the main groups of candidates should be organizations that, because of an inability to recruit nurses, have been unable to participate.

To the extent that some hospices have been unsuccessfully trying to recruit nurses, this provision may enable them to postpone additional efforts and thus save advertising costs. For hospices which have not yet begun to recruit nursing staff, this provision will enable recruitment efforts to be suspended when it can be determined that they will not be effective. We believe that the incremental difference between the incurred costs of current hiring practices and hiring practices of hospices receiving a waiver under this provision will not be significant.

We have determined that this final regulation will not result in a significant economic impact that meets the threshold criteria of Executive Order 12291. In addition, we have determined, and the Secretary certifies that these final regulations will not result in a significant economic impact on a substantial number of small entities. Therefore, we have not prepared either an economic impact analysis or regulatory flexibility analysis.

VI. Information Collection Requirements

Section 418.83(a) of this final rule contains information collection requirements that are subject to Office of Management and Budget (OMB) review under the Paperwork Reduction Act of 1980 (44 U.S.C. 3507). This section has been reviewed by OMB and is approved under OMB No. 0938-0475.

List of Subjects in 42 CFR Part 418

Coinsurance, Hospice, Medicare, Respite care, Volunteers.

For the reasons set forth in the preamble, 42 CFR Part 418 is amended as follows:

PART 418—HOSPICE CARE

1. The authority citation for Part 418 continues to read as follows:

Authority: Secs. 1102, 1811-1814, 1861-1866 and 1871 of the Social Security Act (42 U.S.C. 1302, 1395c-1395f, 1395x-1395cc and 1395hh).

2. Section 418.80 is revised to read as follows:

§ 418.80 Condition of participation—Core services

Except as permitted in § 418.83, a hospice must ensure that substantially all the core services described in §§ 418.82 through 418.88 are routinely provided directly by hospice employees. A hospice may use contracted staff if necessary to supplement hospice employees in order to meet the needs of patients during periods of peak patient loads or under extraordinary circumstances. If contracting is used, the hospice must maintain professional, financial, and administrative responsibility for the services and must assure that the qualifications of staff and services provided meet the requirements specified in §§ 418.82 through 418.88.

3. A new § 418.83 is added to read as follows:

§ 418.83 Nursing services—Waiver of requirement that substantially all nursing services be routinely provided directly by a hospice.

(a) HCFA may approve a waiver of the requirement in § 418.80 for nursing services provided by a hospice which is located in a non-urbanized area. The location of a hospice that operates in several areas is considered to be the location of its central office. The hospice must provide evidence that it was operational on or before January 1, 1983, and that it made a good faith effort to hire a sufficient number of nurses to provide services directly. HCFA bases its decision as to whether to approve a waiver application on the following:

(1) The current Bureau of the Census designations for determining non-urbanized areas.

(2) Evidence that a hospice was operational on or before January 1, 1983 including:

(i) Proof that the organization was established to provide hospice services on or before January 1, 1983;

(ii) Evidence that hospice-type services were furnished to patients on or before January 1, 1983; and

(iii) Evidence that the hospice care was a discrete activity rather than an aspect of another type of provider's patient care program on or before January 1, 1983.

(3) Evidence that a hospice made a good faith effort to hire nurses, including:

(i) Copies of advertisements in local newspapers that demonstrate recruitment efforts;

(ii) Job descriptions for nurse employees;

(iii) Evidence that salary and benefits are competitive for the area; and

(iv) Evidence of any other recruiting activities (e.g., recruiting efforts at health fairs and contacts with nurses at other providers in the area);

(b) Any waiver request is deemed to be granted unless it is denied within 60 days after it is received.

(c) Waivers will remain effective for one year at a time.

(d) HCFA may approve a maximum of two one-year extensions for each initial waiver. If a hospice wishes to receive a one-year extension, the hospice must submit a certification to HCFA, prior to the expiration of the waiver period, that the employment market for nurses has not changed significantly since the time the initial waiver was granted.

(Catalog of Federal Domestic Assistance Program No. 13.773, Medicare Hospital Insurance)

Dated: December 2, 1986.

William L. Roper,
Administrator, Health Care Financing Administration.

Approved: December 31, 1986.

Don M. Newman,
Under Secretary.

[FR Doc. 87-5166 Filed 3-10-87; 8:45 am]

BILLING CODE 4120-01-M

DEPARTMENT OF HEALTH AND HUMAN SERVICES

Health Care Financing Administration

42 CFR Part 418

(BPD-670-FC)

Medicare Program; Hospice Care Amendments: Medicare

AGENCY: Health Care Financing Administration (HCFA), HHS.

ACTION: Final rule with comment period.

SUMMARY: These rules amend the hospice care provisions on physician certification of terminal illness—

• To allow up to 8 days to obtain written certification of terminal illness, provided oral certification is obtained within 2 days after the initial period of care begins; and

• To modify the certification statement which, in its previous form, was shown to discourage physicians from certifying terminal illness and thereby discourage hospice participation in Medicare.

These changes are necessary—

• To conform HCFA rules to amendments made by section 6005(b) of the Omnibus Budget Reconciliation Act of 1989 (OBRA '89); and

• To carry out the recommendations of the General Accounting Office (GAO), aimed at encouraging greater participation of hospices in the Medicare program.

These rules also simplify and clarify other hospice policies, remove outdated content, and correct cross-references.

DATES: *Effective date:* Except for § 418.22, which requires OMB approval before it becomes effective, the rules are effective January 10, 1991.

Comment date: We will consider comments received by February 11, 1991.

ADDRESSES: Please address written comments to: Health Care Financing Administration, Department of Health and Human Services, Attention: BPD-670-FC, P.O. Box 26676, Baltimore, Maryland 21207.

If you prefer, you may deliver your comments to: Room 309—Hubert H. Humphrey Building, 200 Independence Ave., SW., Washington, DC, or Room 132, East High Rise Building, 6325 Security Blvd., Baltimore, Maryland.

Due to staff and resource limitations, we cannot except facsimile (FAX) copies of comments.

In commenting, please refer to file code BPD-670-FC. Comments will be available for public inspection as they are received, beginning approximately 3 weeks from today, in Room 309G of the Department's offices at 200 Independence Ave., SW, Washington, DC on Monday through Friday from 8:30 a.m. to 5 p.m. (202-245-7890).

FOR FURTHER INFORMATION CONTACT: John J. Thomas (301) 966-4623.

SUPPLEMENTARY INFORMATION:

I. Background

Hospice care is an alternative way of treating individuals who are terminally ill. The emphasis in hospice care is on controlling pain and providing services that enable the

---

Source: Reprinted from *Federal Register,* Vol. 55, No. 238, pp. 50831–50835, December 11, 1990.

patient to remain at home as long as possible and to continue normal activities to the extent feasible. Hospices provide social and psychological, as well as medical services. Hospice staff work with the family—helping them to deal with the illness and the anticipated death of the patient. Hospices afford those who are caring for a patient occasional brief periods of respite by providing inpatient care for the beneficiary.

Hospice care emerged in this country around 1975. Medicare coverage of hospice care was established by section 122 of the Tax Equity and Fiscal Responsibility Act of 1982 (Pub. L. 97-248, commonly referred to as "TEFRA"). Since 1983, Medicare beneficiaries certified as terminally ill have had the option of electing hospice care in lieu of most other Medicare-covered services.

A. Statutory Amendment

Section 6005(b) of OBRA '89 (Pub. L. 101-239) amends section 1814(a)(7)(A)(i) of the Act, effective for services furnished on or after January 1, 1990—
• To require that the initial physician certifications of terminal illness be in writing; and
• To allow up to 8 days for the written certifications, provided oral certifications are made within 2 days after the first 90-day period of care begins.

B. Results of GAO Study

After a comprehensive study of the Medicare hospice benefit, GAO found that many physicians were concerned about the statement that they were required to use to certify terminal illness. That statement seemed to require certainty of prognosis, whereas the establishment of long term prognoses always involves some uncertainty. The GAO suggested that physician reluctance to provide certification could be overcome by modifying the statement to incorporate the concept that the certification is based on general knowledge of the normal course of the illness and not on certain knowledge of the patient's prognosis.

II. Changes in the Regulations

1. We have revised § 418.22 of the Medicare rules to reflect both the statutory change and the recommendation that grew out of the GAO study. Specifically—
• Revised paragraph (a) allows up to 8 days after the initial period of care begins for the hospice to obtain written certification of terminal illness provided the hospice obtains oral certification within 2 days.
• Paragraph (b) sets forth the revised certification statement.
• Revised paragraph (c) clarifies which physicians must provide certification for the initial and subsequent periods of care.
• Paragraph (d) requires that hospice staff make appropriate entries in the patient's medical record as soon as they receive oral certifications, and file written certification in that record.

2. We have taken advantage of this opportunity to clarify and simplify the hospice provisions through the following non-substantive changes:
• Undesignated center headings are converted to subpart headings to facilitate references, and several section headings are revised to reflect more accurately the content of the sections.
• Four definitions are removed as unnecessary in these rules. "Carrier" and "Intermediary" are already in the basic definitions at the beginning of the HCFA rules. "Election period" is a matter of rules rather than definition, and this is provided in the new § 418.21.

"Freestanding hospice" was used only in § 418.100 and has been removed as erroneous and misleading, since the requirements of that section apply to all hospices.

• Three definitions have been revised. The previous definition of "Hospice" limited the term to facilities that met all the conditions in part 418. We need a broader definition, since the term is also used in these rules for facilities that do not yet—or no longer—meet all those conditions. The revision of "Representative" is purely editorial, to provide better word order. The revision of "Terminally ill" conforms it to that change made in the required certification statement.

• A new § 418.21 is inserted to substitute for the definition of "Election period" and to set forth the rules for the three periods of hospice care that are available.

• Sections 418.24 and 418.26 are revised to improve readability and combine like requirements within sections.

• Section 418.26 is removed and its content is incorporated in § 418.24.

• Section 418.32 is removed as outdated, and outdated content is removed from §§ 418.98 and 418.204(b)(3).

• Several sections are amended to refer to the newly designated or redesignated subparts.

III. Waiver of Proposed Rulemaking

We ordinarily provide notice and opportunity for public comment before issuing final regulations. The notice of proposed rulemaking (NPRM) identifies the legal authority or the administrative necessity for the proposed rule. It also discusses the substance of, and the reasons for, the particular provisions being proposed. This procedure can be waived when an agency finds that it is impractical, unnecessary, or contrary to the public interest, and incorporates in a final rule a finding of good cause for waiver.

In this particular case, we find that there is good cause to waive NPRM as unnecessary and contrary to the public interest.

We find that notice and opportunity for comments are unnecessary because—

• The statutory amendment is so clear and specific as to leave no room for alternative interpretations.

• Previous rules already require that certifications be in writing; therefore, implementation of the new law actually eases requirements rather than imposing new ones.

• The simplification and clarification of several sections involve no substantive changes.

We also find that it would be contrary to the public interest (as well as the interest of the program) to delay modification of a certification statement that has been shown to discourage the necessary physician certification, and thereby to discourage the participation of hospices in the Medicare program.

Although this rule is final, we will consider any comments received within the time frames specified under "DATES", above. Because of the large number of comments we receive in response to Federal Register publication, we cannot respond to them individually. However, if we revise these rules as a result of comments, we will discuss all timely comments in the preamble to the revised rules.

IV. Regulatory Impact Statement

A. Executive Order 12291

Executive Order 12291 (E.O.12291) requires us to prepare and publish regulatory impact analysis for anyone that meets one of the E.O. 12291 criteria for a "major rule": that is, a rule likely to result in—

• An annual effect on the economy of $100 million or more;

- A major increase in costs or pricing for consumers, individual industries, Federal, State, or local government agencies, or geographic regions.
- Significant adverse effects on competition, employment, or. . . . ability of United States-based enterprises to compete with foreign-based enterprises in domestic or export markets.

Since this rule does not meet any of the E.O. 12291 criteria, a regulatory impact analysis is not required.

B. Regulatory Flexibility Act (RFA)

We generally prepare a regulatory flexibility analysis that is consistent with the Regulatory Flexibility Act (5 U.S.C. 601 through 612) unless the Secretary certifies that a rule will not have a significant economic impact on a substantial number of small entities. For purposes of the RFA, we consider hospices to be small entities.

This final rule extends from 2 to 8 the number of days within which hospices must obtain physician certification of terminal illness, provided the hospice obtains an oral certification within 2 days after the initial period of care begins. This extension should ease the burden on hospices and physicians.

Currently, if a hospice is unable to obtain a written certification within 2 days, the intermediary denies payment for all days of service from the day of admission to the date of certification. With the extension provided under the revised rules (which reflects recommendations made during the GAO survey, as well as the change in the law), hospices should be able to ensure full payment for services furnished to Medicare beneficiaries. This will more than compensate for the very small impact that may result from the requirement that hospice staff note the oral certifications in the patient's medical record.

The GAO report indicated that, as of September, 1989, there were 1,700 hospices in the United States, of which only 35 percent were participating in Medicare. We believe that—

- The extension of time for obtaining written certification of terminal illness will have a favorable economic impact on participating hospices and thus ensure that they will continue to furnish services to Medicare beneficiaries; and
- The cited economic advantage, plus the revised certification statement, which makes it easier to obtain the required physician certifications, will encourage additional hospices to participate in the Medicare program.

Section 1102(b) of the Act requires the Secretary to prepare a regulatory impact analysis for any rule that may have a significant impact on the operations of a substantial number of small rural hospitals. Since this rule applies only to hospices, we have determined and the Secretary certifies that the rule will not have a significant impact on the operations of a substantial number of small rural hospitals.

V. Paperwork Reduction Act

Sections 418.22 and 418.24 of these rules contain information collection requirements that are subject to review by the Office of Management and Budget (OMB) under the Paperwork Reduction Act of 1980. The cited sections had been approved under OMB control number 0938-0246.

Since the certification statement set forth in § 418.22 has been revised, it is again subject to OMB review. When OMB approves the revised statement, we will publish a Federal Register notice to that effect.

If you comment on that revised certification statement, please send a copy of that comment directly to: Office of Information and Regulatory Affairs, Office of Management and Budget, Room 3002, New Executive Office Bldg., Washington, DC 20503, Attention: Allison Herron, Desk Officer for HCFA.

List of Subjects in 42 CFR Part 418

In 42 CFR chapter IV, part 418 is amended as set forth below:
A.1. The authority citation for part 418 continues to read as follows:
Authority: Secs. 1102, 1811-1814, 1815(e), 1861-1866, and 1871 of the Social Security Act (42 U.S.C. 1302, 1395c-1395f, 1395g(e), 1395x-1395cc, and 1395hh).
2. The table of contents is revised to read as follows:

PART 418—HOSPICE CARE

Subpart A—General Provisions and Definitions

Sec.
418.1 Statutory basis.
418.2 Scope of part.
418.3 Definitions.

Subpart B—Eligibility, Election and Duration of Benefits

418.20 Eligibility requirements.
418.21 Duration of hospice care coverage—Election periods.
418.22 Certification of terminal illness.
418.24 Election of hospice care.
418.28 Revoking the election of hospice care.
418.30 Change of the designated hospice.

Subpart C—Conditions of Participation, General Provisions and Administration

418.50 Condition of participation—General provisions.
418.52 Condition of participation—Governing body.
418.54 Condition of participation—Medical director.
418.56 Condition of participation—Professional management.
418.58 Condition of participation—Plan of care.
418.60 Condition of participation—Continuation of care.
418.62 Condition of participation—Informed consent.
418.64 Condition of participation—Inservice training.
418.66 Condition of participation—Quality assurance.
418.68 Condition of participation—Interdisciplinary group.
418.70 Condition of participation—Volunteers.
418.72 Condition of participation—Licensure.
418.74 Condition of participation—Central clinical records.

Subpart D—Condition of participation: Core Services

418.80 Condition of participation—Furnishing of core services.
418.82 Condition of participation—Nursing services.

418.83 Condition of participation—Nursing services—Waiver of requirement that substantially all nursing services be routinely provided directly by a hospice.
418.84 Condition of participation—Medical social services.
418.86 Condition of participation—Physician services.
418.88 Condition of participation—Counseling services.

Subpart E—Conditions of participation. Other Services

418.90 Condition of participation—Furnishing of other services.
418.92 Condition of participation—Physical therapy, occupational therapy, and speech-language pathology.
418.94 Condition of participation—Home health aide and homemaker services.
418.96 Conditions of participation—Medical supplies.
418.98 Condition of participation—Short term inpatient care.
418.100 Condition of participation—Hospices that provide inpatient care directly.

Subpart F—Covered Services

418.200 Requirements for coverage.
418.202 Covered services.
418.204 Special coverage requirements.

Subpart G—Payment for Hospice Care

418.301 Reimbursement for hospice care.
418.302 Payment procedures for hospice care.
418.304 Payment for physician services.
418.306 Determination of payment rates.
418.307 Periodic interim payments.
418.308 Limitation on the amount of hospice payments.
418.309 Hospice cap amount.
418.310 Reporting and recordkeeping requirements.
418.311 Administrative appeals.

Subpart H—Coinsurance

418.400 Individual liability for coinsurance for hospice care.
418.402 Individual liability for services that are not considered hospice care.
418.405 Reduction of Medicare reimbursement by individual coinsurance liability.

3. Subparts D, E, and F are redesignated as subparts F, G, and H, respectively.
B. Subpart A is amended as follows:

Subpart A—General Provisions and Definitions

§ 418.3 (Amended)

In § 418.3, the definitions of *"Carrier"*, *"Election period"*, *"Freestanding hospice"*, and *"Intermediary"* are removed and the definitions of *"Hospice"*, *"Representative"*, and *"Terminally ill"* are revised to read as follows:

Hospice means a public agency or private organization or subdivision of either of these that—is primarily engaged in providing care to terminally ill individuals.

* * * * *

Representative means an individual who has been authorized under State law to terminate medical care or to elect or revoke the election of hospice care on behalf of a terminally ill individual who is mentally or physically incapacitated.

* * * * *

Terminally ill means that the individual has a medical prognosis that his or her life expectancy is 6 months or less if the illness runs its normal course.

C. Subpart B is amended as follows:

Subpart B—Eligibility, Election and Duration of Benefits

1. A new § 418.21 is added, to read as follows:

§ 418.21 Duration of hospice care coverage—Election periods.

(a) Subject to the conditions set forth in this part, an individual may elect to receive hospice care during one or more of the following election periods:

(1) An initial 90-day period.

(2) A subsequent 90-day period.

(3) A subsequent 30-day period.

(b) The periods of care are available in the order listed and may be elected separately at different times.

§ 418.22 (Amended)

2. Section 418.22 is revised to read as follows:

§ 418.22 Certification of terminal illness.

(a) *Timing of certification—*

(1) *General rule.* The hospice must obtain written certification of terminal illness for each of the periods listed in § 418.21, even if a single election continues in effect for two or three periods, as provided in § 418.24(c).

(2) *Basic requirement.* Except as provided in paragraph (a)(3) of this section, the hospice must obtain the written certification no later than two calendar days after the period begins.

(3) *Exception.* For the initial 90-day period, if the hospice cannot obtain the written certifications within two calendar days, it must obtain oral certifications within two calendar days, and written certifications no later than eight calendar days after the period begins.

(b) *Consent of certification.* Thus certification must specify that the individual's prognosis is for a life expectancy of 6 months or less if the terminal illness runs its normal course.

(c) *Sources of certification.*

(1) For the initial 90-day period, the hospice must obtain written certification statements (and oral certification statements if required under paragraph (a)(3) of this section) from—

(i) The medical director of the hospice or the physician member of the hospice interdisciplinary group; and

(ii) The individual's attending physician if the individual has an attending physician.

(2) For subsequent periods, the only requirement is certification by one of the physicians listed in paragraph (c)(1)(i) of this section.

(d) *Maintenance of records.* Hospice staff must—

(1) Make an appropriate entry in the patient's medical record as soon as they receive an oral certification; and

(2) File written certification in the medical record.

§ 418.24 (Amended)

3. Section 418.24 for his revised to read as follows:

418.24 Election of hospice care.

(a) *Filing an election statement.* An individual who meets the eligibility requirements of § 418.20 may file an election statement with a particular hospice. If the individual is physically or mentally incapacitated, his or her representative (as defined in § 418.3) may file the election statement.

(b) *Consent of election statement.* The election statement must include the following:

(1) Identification of the particular hospice that will provide care to the individual.

(2) The individual's or representative's acknowledgement that he or she has been given a full understanding of the palliative rather than curative nature of hospice care, as it relates to the individual's terminal illness.

(3) Acknowledgement that certain Medicare services, as set forth in paragraph (d) of this section, are waived by the election.

(4) The effective date of the election, which may be the first day of hospice care or a later date, but may be no earlier than the date of the election statement.

(5) The signature of the individual or representative.

(c) *Duration of election.* An election to receive hospice care will be considered to continue through the initial election period and through the subsequent election periods without a break in care as long as the individual—

(1) Remains in the care of a hospice; and

(2) Does not revoke the election under the provisions of § 418.28.

(d) *Waiver of other benefits.* For the duration of an election of hospice care, an individual waives all rights to Medicare payments for the following services:

(1) Hospice care provided by a hospice other than the hospice designated by the individual (unless provided under arrangements made by the designated hospice).

(2) Any Medicare services that are related to the treatment of the terminal condition for which hospice care was elected or a related condition or that are equivalent to hospice care except for services—

(i) Provided by the designated hospice:

(ii) Provided by another hospice under arrangements made by the designated hospice; and

(iii) Provided by the individual's attending physician if that physician is not an employee of the designated hospice or receiving compensation from the hospice for those services.

(e) *Re-election of hospice benefits.* If an election has been revoked in accordance with § 418.28, the individual (or his or her representative if the individual is mentally or physically incapacitated) may at any time following an election, in accordance with this section, for any other election period that is still available to the individual.

§ 418.26 (Removed)

4. Section 418.26 is removed.

§ 418.32 (Removed)

5. Section 418.32 is removed.
D. Subpart C is amended as set forth below:
1. The subpart heading is revised and § 418.50(a) is revised, to read as follows:

Subpart C—Conditions of Participation—General Provisions and Administration

§ 418.50 Conditions of participation—General provisions.

(a) *Standard: Compliance.* A hospice must maintain compliance with the conditions of this subpart and subparts D and E of this part.

* * * * *

2. The undesignated center heading "Administration" is removed.
3. The undesignated center heading " Core Services" is revised to read as follows:

Subpart D—Conditions of Participation: Core Services

§ 418.80 (Amended)

4. In § 418.80, the following changes are made:
a. Thus section heading is revised to read:

§ 418.80 Condition of participation: Furnishing of core services.

b. The phrase "§§ 418.82 through 418.88", wherever it appears, is changed to "this subpart".
5. The undesignated center heading "Other Services" is revised to read:

Subpart E—Conditions of Participation: Other Services

§ 418.90 (Amended)

6. In § 418.90, the following changes are made:
a. The section heading is revised to read:

§ 418.90 Condition of participation: Furnishing of other services.

b. The phrase "§§ 418.92 to 418.93" is changed to "this subpart".

§ 418.94 (Amended)

7. In § 418.94, the following changes are made:
a. In the introductory text to the section, "§ 405.1227" is changed to "§ 484.36".
b. In paragraph (b), "§ 405.1227(a)" is changed to "§ 484.36(c)".

§ 418.98 (Amended)

8. In § 418.98, the following changes are made:

a. In paragraphs (a)(2) and (b)(2), "(f)" is changed to "(e)".

b. Paragraph (c) is revised to read as follows:

(c) *Standard: Inpatient care limitation.* The total number of inpatient days used by Medicare beneficiaries who elected hospice coverage in any 12-month period preceding a certification survey in a particular hospice may not exceed 20 percent of the total number of hospice days for this group of beneficiaries.

9. The undesignated center heading "Freestanding Hospice with Inpatient Unit" is removed.

§ 418.100 (Amended)

10. In § 418.100, the following changes are made:

a. The section heading is revised to read:

§ 418.100 Condition of participation: Hospices that provide inpatient care directly.

b. The word "freestanding" is removed from the introductory text.

E. Newly redesignated subpart F is amended as follows:

§ 418.202 (Amended)

1. In § 418.202, in paragraph (e), "§ 418.100 (a) and (f)" is changed to "§ 418.202 (a) and (e)".

§ 418.204 (Amended)

2. Section 418.204 is amended by revising paragraph (b)(2) and removing paragraph (b)(3), to read as follows:

§ 418.204 Special coverage requirements.

* * * * *

(b) *Respite care.*

(1) Respite care is short-term inpatient care provided to the individual only when necessary to relieve the family members or other persons caring for the individual.

(2) Respite care may be provided only on an occasional basis and may not be reimbursed for more than five consecutive days at a time.

* * * * *

F. Newly redesignated subpart G is amended by revising the subpart heading to read as follows:

Subpart G—Payment for hospice care

(Catalog of Federal Domestic Assistance Programs No. 13.773, Medicare Hospital Insurance)

Dated: June 5, 1990.

Gail R. Wilensky,
Administrator, Health Care Financing Administration.

Approved: July 9, 1990.

Louis W. Sullivan,
Secretary.

(FR Doc. 90-28756 Filed 12-10-90; 8:45 am)

BILLING CODE 4120-01-M

PROGRAM MEMORANDUM

INTERMEDIARIES

Department of Health and Human Services

Health Care Financing Administration

Transmittal No. A-98-27 Date: SEPTEMBER 1998

Change Request #N/A

This Program Memorandum re-releases Program Memorandum A-97-11, dated September 1997. Changes are redlined.

SUBJECT: Hospice Provisions Enacted by the Balanced Budget Act (BBA) of 1997

The purpose of this Program Memorandum is to clarify recent legislation enacted by the BBA of 1997 as it applies to Medicare hospice services and provide guidance on billing instructions for these services. Many of these provisions were effective upon enactment of the legislation; that is, August 5, 1997. These changes are a result of a Congressional mandate, and should be made immediately. Providers should be billing for those services based on the changes described below.

A. Payment For Home Hospice Care Based On Location Where Care Is Furnished.—The BBA of 1997 requires that hospices submit claims for payment for hospice care furnished in an individual's home (i.e., revenue codes 651 and 652) based on the geographic location at which the service is furnished (as opposed to the location of the hospice). HCFA is in the process of developing a pricing system that will be used by the fiscal intermediaries which will determine the rate for these services. Providers will be required to indicate the metropolitan statistical area (MSA)/rural state code number with value code 61 on the bill.

1. Fiscal Intermediary Instructions.—For dates of service beginning on or after October 1, 1997, reject hospice claims bill types 81X and 82X with revenue codes 651 (routine home care) and 652 (continuous home care) that do not contain value code 61 (where the service is delivered) and an MSA (Metropolitan Statistical Area) code/rural state code. A table identifying the appropriate MSA for each location is attached. Only revenue codes 651 and 652 require the value code and MSA for site of service.

Edit the claim for the presence and the validity of the MSA code. The MSA code for hospice claims is a 4 or 5 digit field. The common working file will also reject home care claims that do not contain value code 61 and a MSA beginning October 1 for revenue codes 651 and 652.

2. Coding Requirements.—

• Show value code 61 for home care revenue codes (651 and 652) and enter the MSA (a 4 or 5 digit numerical).

• On the UB92 rev. 4.1, show the value code and MSA in Record Type 41 fields 16–39. There can be up to 12 occurrences.

Since the value amount is a nine-position field, enter the 4–5 MSA code in the nine-position field in the following manner: Enter an MSA for Puerto Rico as 000994000 and the MSA for Abilene TX (0040) as 000004000. Note that the two characters to the right of the assumed decimal point (9999999V99) are always zeros.

Source: Reprinted from http://www.hcfa.gov.

• To create parallel construction for the electronic X12 institutional claim transaction (837 Medicare version 3032 and 3051) and the electronic UB-92, use the HI segment to contain MSA data. For example, enter an MSA of 9940 as 000994000 on the electronic UB-92; this would be translated as HI*BE:61:::9940~. For the MSA of 0040, enter 000004000 on the electronic UB-92 and translate this as HI*BE:61:::40~. Note that this constuction permits our current maps to work without change.

• On the HCFA 1450, in field location 39–41, show value code 61 in the code area and the 4–5 position MSA in the amount area where a dollar amount could be entered.

Do not extend the MSA into the cents area.

Send the above information to all hospices in your provider file, to hospice professional groups, and software support organizations.

B. Hospice Care Benefit Periods.—The BBA of 1997 restructured the hospice benefit periods available to Medicare beneficiaries as provided for under §1812 of the Social Security Act (the Act). Effective upon the date of enactment, August 5, 1997, the hospice benefit has two initial 90-day periods followed by an unlimited number of subsequent 60-day periods. Each period requires a physician to certify at the beginning of the period that the individual has a terminal illness with a prognosis that the individual's life expectancy is 6 months or less. 42 CFR 418.22(b) clarifies that a physician's certification specifies that the prognosis is for a life expectancy of 6 months or less, but qualifies it with the words "if the terminal illness runs its normal course," recognizing that such a prognosis is not entirely predictable. This provision of the regulation remains unchanged.

The change in the law affects certain beneficiaries in the former third period of 30 days and the fourth period of unlimited duration. On the date of enactment, these periods essentially "disappeared." Consequently, beneficiaries in their third period will be automatically considered in their first subsequent period of 60 days. The period will be considered to have begun on the date of enactment. Recertification will be required at the beginning of the next 60-day period and for every 60-day period thereafter as may be indicated. Beneficiaries in their fourth period will be considered as having begun their first 60-day period as of the date of enactment (August 5, 1997) and the first recertification will be required at the beginning of the next 60-day period, and for every 60-day period thereafter as may be indicated.

Section 4449 of the BBA of 1997 indicated that the benefit period changes applied to the hospice benefit regardless of whether or not an individual had made an election of the benefit prior to the date of enactment. Therefore, a beneficiary who elected hospice prior to the BBA of 1997 and who may be discharged from hospice care at some future time because he or she is no longer terminally ill could avail themselves of the benefit at some later date if they should become terminally ill again and otherwise meet the requirements of the Medicare hospice benefit. If the beneficiary had been discharged during the initial 90-day period, he or she would enter the benefit in the second 90-day period. If the discharge took place during the final 90-day or any subsequent 60-day period, the beneficiary would enter the benefit in a new 60-day period. A beneficiary who had been discharged from hospice during the fourth benefit period prior to the enactment of the BBA of 1997 would be eligible for the benefit again and would begin it in a 60-day period. The 90-day periods would not be available as the amended §1812(d)(1) of the Act still only provides for two 90-day periods during an individual's lifetime. There is no limit on 60-day periods as long as the beneficiary meets the requirements for the hospice benefit.

With respect to the changes in the benefit period structure, HCFA will accept corrected certfication statements in cases of billing errors. Other changes in physician certification requirements are discussed in another section below.

C. Other Items And Services.—A new item has been added to the list of covered services in §1861(dd)(1) of the Act. The new item "I" explains that any other item or service which is specified in the plan and for which payment may otherwise be made under this title is a covered service under the Medicare hospice benefit. This new item is a clarification of past policy that the hospice is responsible for providing any and all services indicated as necessary for the palliation and management of the terminal illness and related conditions in the plan of care.

EXAMPLE: A hospice determines that a patient's condition has worsened and has become medically unstable. An inpatient stay will be necessary for proper palliation and management of the condition. The hospice adds this inpatient stay to the plan of care and decides that, due to the patient's fragile condition, the patient will need to be transported to the hospital by ambulance. In this case, the ambulance service becomes a covered hospice service.

This clarification becomes effective for items or services furnished on or after April 1, 1998.

D. Contracting With Physicians.—The BBA of 1997 also includes a provision that amends the core service requirement to allow hospices to contract for physician services. Effective August 5, 1997, §1861(dd)(2) of the Act is amended so that hospices will no longer be required to routinely provide all physician services directly.

Medical directors and physician members of the interdisciplinary group (IDG) are no longer required to be employed by the hospice. These physicians can now be "under contract" with the hospice. Although Congress did not specify what the terms of that contract must be, requirements at 42 CFR 418.56 and 418.86 are still applicable to hospice, as well as all other responsibilities under the hospice conditions of participation. Hospices retain professional management responsibilities for these services and must ensure that they are furnished in a safe and effective manner by qualified persons.

E. Waiver Of Certain Staffing Requirements.—Section 1861(dd)(5) of the Act has been modified to allow HCFA to permit certain waivers of the requirements that the hospice make physical therapy, occupational therapy, speech language pathology services, and dietary counseling available (as needed) on a 24-hour basis. HCFA is also now allowed to waive the requirement that hospices provide dietary counseling directly. These waivers are available only to an agency or organization that is located in an area which is not an urbanized area (as defined by the Bureau of Census) and that can demonstrate to HCFA that it has been unable, despite diligent efforts, to recruit appropriate personnel. Hospices will be required to submit evidence to establish "diligent efforts." HCFA will apply the requirements for the nursing services waiver found at 42 CFR 418.83(a)(3) in determining that a hospice has made diligent efforts. A waiver request will be deemed to be granted unless it is denied within 60 days after it is received. This change became effective upon enactment of the Balanced Budget Act, or August 5, 1997. Waiver applications should be sent to your regional office.

F. Limitation On Liability Of Beneficiaries For Certain Hospice Coverage Denials—Section 1879 of the Act provides protections from liability for charges for certain denied claims to beneficiaries who, acting in good faith, receive inpatient or outpatient services from Medicare Part A providers, or items or services from Medicare Part B suppliers which accept assignment. Likewise, providers and suppliers may also be protected from liability under §1879 of the Act when it is determined that they did not know and could not reasonably have been expected to know that Medicare would deny payment. When the beneficiary is held not liable and the provider also is held to be not liable, payment may be made for a denied claim under §1879, as if the service were covered. Section 1879(g) of the

Act has been amended by §4447 of the BBA of 1997 to extend limitation on liability protection to a beneficiary enrolled in a hospice when there is a denial of claims due to a determination that the individual is not terminally ill. Effective for services furnished on or after August 5, 1997, when a denial of payment for hospice services is based upon a determination that the beneficiary is not terminally ill, apply the usual procedures of the limitation on liability provision under §3430ff of the Medicare Intermediary Manual (MIM), and (as appropriate) the indemnification procedures under §3446ff of the MIM, to determine whether or not the beneficiary is protected from liability, and whether or not the hospice is protected from liability, under §1879(g)(2) of the Act.

G. Extending The Period For Physician Certification Of An Individual's Terminal Illness.—The BBA of 1997 amended §1814(a)(7)(A)(i) of the Act by removing specific written and verbal time frames for physician certifications (that an individual is terminally ill) for the initial 90-day benefit period and requiring only that certification be done "at the beginning of the period". Certification by physicians for hospice care at the beginning of the initial benefit period will remain as they are currently, i.e., "beginning of the period" continues to be not later that 2 days after hospice care begins, but written certification need only be on file in the patient's record prior to submission of a claim to the fiscal intermediary. An initial plan of care must be established at the start of care, prepared by the hospice physician or nurse, in consultation with the attending physician (if there is one) or the hospice physician if there is no attending physician and one other member of the IDG.

This requirement would apply to individuals who had been previously discharged during a fourth benefit period and were being certified for hospice care again to begin care in a 60-day benefit period. As had been discussed in a 1995 Bulletin For Hospice Providers, certifications of terminal illness must include specific clinical findings and other documentation supporting a life expectancy of 6 months or less.

For policy questions, contact Jennifer Carter (410) 786-4615, Tom Saltz (410) 786-4480, or Carol Blackford (410) 786-5909.

For questions relating to the conditions of participation, contact Lynn Merritt-Nixon (410) 786-4652 or Mary Vienna (410) 786-6940.

For questions relating to limitation on liability, contact Joan Collins (410) 786-4618 or Denis Garrison (410) 786-5643.

For questions concerning fiscal intermediary instructions and coding, contact Pat Williams (410) 786-6139.

This Program Memorandum may be discarded after September 1, 1999.

These instructions should be implemented within our current operating budget.

INDEX

A

Abbreviations, xv
Abington Memorial Hospital Compliance Program, 4–5
Abington Memorial Hospital, bylaws, 17–25
   amendments, 25
   Board of Trustees, 17–19
   chief of staff, 24
   committees, 20–23
   indemnification, 24
   medical, dental, and podiatric staff, 23–24
   membership, 17
   officers, 19–20
   purpose, 17
Abuse, 135–137
   policy, 135–136
   procedure, 136–137
Acquired immune deficiency syndrome. *See* AIDS
Acronyms, xv
Admission criteria, 8–9
   policy, 8–9
Advance directive
   policy, 9–10
   procedure, 10–12
Adverse drug reaction, medication, 95
AIDS
   policy, 12–13
   procedures, 13–15
Annual administrative review, form, 144
Annual competencies, 38

B

Balanced Budget Act, xiii, 258–261
Bereavement counseling program, 43, 219
   characteristics, 15–16
   policy, 15
   procedure, 16
   volunteer, 15–16
   training, 16
Bereavement risk, assessment form, 145, 146
Bereavement service, follow-up form, 147
Bibliography, xiii
Board of Trustees, 17–19
   conditions of participation, 208
   hospice, 58

C

Care level, 87–88
   continuous care, 87
   inpatient care
      acute, 88
      respite, 88
   policy, 87–88
   routine home care, 87
Care plan, form, 166
Carrier, 224–226
Centers for Disease Control, infection control, 74
Certification of staff
   home health aide, 62–68
      procedure, 63–68
   verification, 88–89
Certification of terminal illness, 206
   amendment, 247–251, 253–254, 261
Certification of terminal illness statement, 8
Clinical record, 5–6, 25–31
   completion, 34
   computer mail documentation, 34
   conditions of participation, 212
   confidentiality, 33
   consent for release of information form, 149
   discharged patient, 31–32
   filing sequence, 154
   master file input data, 26–27
   open records, 26–31
   policy, 26
   procedure, 26–34

protection of records, 33
record documentation, 32–33
release, 33–34
    HIV information, 119–120
reopening previous admission, 31
Coinsurance, 223–224
    individual liability, 223
        reduction of Medicare reimbursement, 223–224
Communication, 65–66
    emergency preparedness plan, 52–53
    hearing impaired patient, 36–37
        policy, 36
        procedure, 36–37
    language interpreter, 34–35
    non-English language speaking patient, 34–35
    visually impaired patient, 36–37
        policy, 36
        procedure, 36–37
Competency evaluation program, 37–40
    home health aide, 62–68
    policy, 37–38
    procedure, 38–40
Compliance Program, 4–5
    Employee Hotline, 4–5
    standards, 4
Conditions of participation
    clinical record, 212
    continuation of care, 210
    core services, 212
        amendments, 255–257
    counseling, 213
    cross-references, 199–200
    freestanding hospice with inpatient unit, 214–217
    general provisions, 208
    governing body, 208
    home health aide, 213–214
    homemaker services, 213–214
    informed consent, 210
    inpatient care, short term, 214
    interdisciplinary group, 210–211
    licensure, 211
    medical director, 208
    medical social services, 212
    medical supplies, 214
    nursing services, 212
    occupational therapy, 213
    physical therapy, 213
    physician, 213
    plan of care, 209–210
    professional management, 209
    quality assurance, 210
    speech-language pathology services, 213
    training, 210
    volunteer, 211
Confidentiality
    clinical record, 33
    consent for release of information form, 149
Conflict of interest, 40–42
    policy, 41
    procedure, 41–42
Consultation, 41
    medical social work, 126
    occupational therapy, 104

physical therapy, 113
speech pathology services, 128
Continuous care, 87
Controlled drug, disposal, 47–48
Counseling, 43
    conditions of participation, 213

D

Death pronouncement, registered nurse, 44–46
    policy, 44–45
    procedure, 45–46
Disaster, definition, 52
Discharge, 47
    hospice discharge checklist
        inpatient care, 157–158, 159–160
            routine services, 159–160, 161–162
    requirements, 47
    summary, 27–28
Do not resuscitate (DNR), 10, 11, 49–50, 140
    policy, 49
    procedure, 49–50
Documentation
    medical social work, 126
    occupational therapy, 104–105
    physical therapy, 113–114
    speech pathology services, 128–129
Durable medial equipment, reporting procedures, 89

E

Eligibility, 202, 205–206
Emergency, definition, 52
Emergency phone numbers, 51
Emergency preparedness plan, 51–54
    communication, 52–53
    policy, 51
    procedure, 52–53
Employee assistance program, stress management, 71
Employee Hotline, Compliance Program, 4–5
Engineering and work practice controls, exposure control plan, 55
Entitlement, 202
Entry-level competencies, 38
Ethical issues, 6–7
    policy, 6–7
    procedure, 7
Ethical nursing practice model, 6
Exposure control plan, 54–58
    communication of hazards to employees, 57
    compliance methods, 54–55
    effective dates, 57–58
    engineering and work practice controls, 55
    exposure classification, 54
    exposure determination, 54
    handwashing, 55
    hepatitis B vaccination, 55–56
    personal protective equipment, 55
    policy, 54
    postexposure evaluation and follow-up, 56–57
    universal precautions, 54–55

F

Federal Register, 201–261
Funeral director, letter of explanation for, 86–87
Furosemide, 98

G

Gloves, 75–76
Governing body, conditions of participation, 208
Grief recovery support group, 16

H

Handwashing, 75
    exposure control plan, 55
Hearing impaired patient, communication, 36–37
    policy, 36
    procedure, 36–37
Hepatitis B vaccination, 55–56
Home care services, 58–59
Home health aide, 43, 59–62
    certification, 62–68
        procedure, 63–68
    competency evaluation program, 62–68
        policy, 62–63
        procedure, 63–68
    conditions of participation, 213–214
    policy, 60
    procedure, 60–62
    training, 62–68
        policy, 62–63
        procedure, 63–68
Home visit consent form, 163
Homemaker services, 43, 59–62
    conditions of participation, 213–214
    policy, 60
    procedure, 60–62
Hospice
    board of trustees, 58
    change of designated hospice, 207
    core services, 42–44
    core services waiver requirements, 241–243
    election of hospice benefit
        amendments, 254
        informed consent form, 152
    goals, 116
    governing body, 58
    introduction, 238
    legislative history, 238–239
    non-urbanized areas, 239–246
    nursing services requirement waiver, 239–246
    organizational chart, 107
    organizational mission, 108
    personal care facility, 70–71
        policy, 70
        procedure, 70–71
    program statement, 114
    purpose, 116
    skilled nursing facility, 70–71
        policy, 70
        procedure, 70–71
Hospice support group
    interdisciplinary group, 71
    stress management, 71
Hospital ethics committee, 7
Housekeeping, 79–80

I

Imferon, 97
Incident reporting, 72–74
    departmental incident report tracking form, 151
    form, 150
    medication, 95
    policy, 72
    procedure, 72–74
Indemnification, 24
Infection control
    Centers for Disease Control, 74
    Occupational Safety and Health Act, 74
    tracking and reporting, 81–82
        policy, 81–82
        procedure, 82
    universal blood and body fluid precautions, 74–81
        communication of hazards to employees, 80–81
        contaminated sharps, 77–78
        equipment, 79
        housekeeping, 79–80
        lab specimens, 78–79
        laundry, 80
        policy, 74
        post-contact cleansing requirements, 77
        pregnancy, 81
        procedure, 75
Informed consent
    conditions of participation, 210
    patient consent for care form, 177
Inpatient care
    acute, form, 143
    care level, 88
    conditions of participation, short term, 214
    respite care, 44
    plan of care, 179
    symptom control, 43–44
    volunteer, 68–70
Intake procedure, 82–84
Interdisciplinary care plan, 86
    form, 166
Interdisciplinary group
    conditions of participation, 210–211
    coordination, 85
    form, 166
    hospice support group, 71
    members, ix
    policy, 84–85
    policy approval, ix
    policy development, viii
    policy review, ix
Intermediary, 224–226
    change to another intermediary, 225
    change to direct payment, 225
    defined, 225

designation for freestanding home health agencies
    and hospices, 226
hearing, 226
nominations, 225
right to judicial review, 226

L

Lab specimens, 78–79
Language interpreter, 34–35
    policy, 35
    procedure, 35
Laundry, 80
Licensure, 39
    conditions of participation, 211
        verification, 88–89
            physician, 134–135
Life-sustaining care withdrawal, 139–140

M

Medical device, reporting procedures, 89
Medical director, conditions of participation, 208
Medical record. *See* Clinical record
Medical services plan of care, 90–92
    policy, 91
    procedures, 91–92
Medical social services, 124–126
    competency, in-home evaluation form, 167–168
    conditions of participation, 212
    consultation, 126
    documentation, 126
    policy, 125
    procedure, 125–126
Medical supplies, 43
    conditions of participation, 214
Medicare
    benefits, 202
    change of designated hospice, 207
    core services waiver requirements, 241–243
    corrections, 228–237
    covered services, 218–219
    definitions, 205
    duration of coverage, 208
    election of hospice care, 50
        elements of election statement, 207
        informed consent form, 152
        revoking, 206–207, 207
    eligibility requirements, 50–51
    limitation on liability of beneficiaries for certain
        hospice coverage denials, 260–261
    non-urbanized areas, 239–246
    physician certification/recertification of terminal
        illness form, 178
    program integrity, 224
    reimbursement, 219–223
        administrative appeals, 222–223
        based on location where care is furnished, 258–259
        benefits period, 259
        cap amount, 222
        limitation on amount of payments, 222

payment procedures, 219–221
payment rate determination, 221–222
physician services, 221
reporting and recordkeeping requirements, 222
requirements for coverage, 218
revoking election of hospice care, 50–51
    form, 164
social services, 42–43
waiver of certain staffing requirements, 260
waiver of nursing services requirement, 239–246
Medication, 93–99
    administration, 93–94
    adverse drug reaction, 95
    drugs given for research purposes, 98–99
    errors, 96
    incident report, 95
    intramuscular/subcutaneous/intravenous
        administration, 96–98
    policy, 93
    procedure, 93–99
    self-administration, 93
    supervision, 94–95
    teaching, 94–95
    unlabeled drugs, 96
Medication list, 27

N

Neglect, 135–137
    policy, 135–136
    procedure, 136–137
Non-English language speaking patient,
    communication, 34–35
Nursing, competency, in-home evaluation form, 169–170
Nursing assessment form, 27
Nursing services, 42, 99–102
    conditions of participation, 212
    non-patient care, 101–102
    patient care, 100–101
    policy, 100
    procedure, 100–102
    quality assurance, 180–184
    quarterly record review, 180–184
    services not permitted, 102
    waiver for non-urbanized areas, 239–246
Nutrition counseling, 43

O

Occupational Safety and Health Act, infection control, 74
Occupational therapy, 43, 102–105
    competency, in-home evaluation form, 194–195
    conditions of participation, 213
    consultation, 104
    documentation, 104–105
    policy, 103
    procedure, 103–105
    supervision, 104
Organizational chart, 107

Organizational mission, 108
Orientation, 108–109
   hospice contractor orientation program form, 155–156
   policy, 109
   procedure, 109
   staff, form, 171–174
Outside employment, 41

P

Pain and symptom management, 110
Pain assessment form, 175–176
Pastoral care, 43
   operational agreement, 105–106
Patient consent for care, 8–9
Patient Self-Determination Act, 9–12
Patient's bill of rights/responsibilities, 110–111
Patient's representative, 9
Penicillin, 97
Personal care facility, hospice, 70–71
   policy, 70
   procedure, 70–71
Personal protective equipment, 76–77
   exposure control plan, 55
Physical therapy, 43, 111–114
   conditions of participation, 213
   consultation, 113
   documentation, 113–114
   policy, 112
   procedure, 112–114
   supervision, 113
Physician, 42
   conditions of participation, 213
   contracting with, 261
   licensure, verification, 134–135
   plan of treatment, 27
Plan of care, 86
   conditions of participation, 209–210
   in-patient respite care, 179
   medical services, 90–92
Policy
   approval process, viii
      conditions of participation, viii
   areas of nursing needing, vii
   components, vii
   defined, vii
   need for, vii
   review, viii
      conditions of participation, viii
Policy development, viii
   interdisciplinary group, viii
   personnel involved, viii
Postorientation/probationary competencies, 38
Pregnancy, 81
Primary care person, 8–9
Professional advisory committee, viii
Provider
   agreements under Medicare, 226–227
   defined, 225
   options available to, 225
Psychiatric counseling, 43

Q

Quality assessment and improvement program, 116–117
   methods, 117
   objectives, 117
   policy, 116
Quality assurance
   conditions of participation, 210
   nursing services, 180–184
Quarterly record review, 117, 118
   nursing services, 180–184

R

Readings on death, dying, bereavement, resource list, 187–192
Reference check, 38–39
Referral, between hospital and hospice, 115–116
Registered nurse, death pronouncement, 44–46
   policy, 44–45
   procedure, 45–46
Reimbursement, Medicare, 219–223
   administrative appeals, 222–223
   based on location where care is furnished, 258–259
   benefits period, 259
   cap amount, 222
   limitation on amount of payments, 222
   payment procedures, 219–221
   payment rate determination, 221–222
   physician services, 221
   reporting and recordkeeping requirements, 222
Religious assessment form, 193
Resource list
   readings on death, dying, bereavement, 187–192
   religious group, 185–186
Respite care, 28, 219
   care level, 88
   inpatient care, 44

S

Safe Medical Device Act, 89
Safety standards, 120–121
   policy, 121
   procedure, 121–122
Skilled nursing facility, hospice, 70–71
   policy, 70
   procedure, 70–71
Social worker, 42–43
Solganal, 97–98
Speech pathology services, 43, 127–129
   conditions of participation, 213
   consultation, 128
   policy, 127
   procedure, 127–129
Spiritual assessment form, 193
Staff development, 129–131
   policy, 130
   procedure, 130–131
Staff evaluation, 122–124
   policy, 122

procedure, 122–124
Staff orientation, 122–124
   form, 171–174
   policy, 122
   procedure, 122–124
Staff selection, 122–124
   policy, 122
   procedure, 122–124
Standards, 4
Stress management
   employee assistance program, 71
   hospice support group, 71
Supervision
   medication, 94–95
   occupational therapy, 104
   physical therapy, 113
Support group, for hospice team members, 131
Syringe, used syringe disposal, 48–49

T

Teaching, medication, 94–95
Terminal Care Fund, 5
Training
   conditions of participation, 210
   home health aide, 62–68
     policy, 62–63
     procedure, 63–68
   volunteer
     bereavement syllabus, 165
     program syllabus, 197
Transfer, 131–132
   change of designated hospice form, 148
   form, 153
Twenty-four-hour service, 132–133
   policy, 132–133
   procedure, 133

U

Uniform Determination of Death Act, 45
Universal blood and body fluid precautions
   exposure control plan, 54–55
   infection control, 74–81
     communication of hazards to employees, 80–81
     contaminated sharps, 77–78
     equipment, 79
     housekeeping, 79–80
     lab specimens, 78–79
     laundry, 80
     policy, 74
     post-contact cleansing requirements, 77
     pregnancy, 81
     procedure, 75
Utilization review, 117, 134

V

Violence, 135–137
   policy, 135–136
   procedure, 136–137
Visually impaired patient, communication, 36–37
   policy, 36
   procedure, 36–37
Volunteer, 68–70, 138–139
   assessment and plan: inpatient unit form, 196
   assignment form, 196
   bereavement program, 15–16
     training, 16
   conditions of participation, 211
   inhospital patient, 68–70
   policy, 69, 138
   procedure, 69–70, 138–139
   recruitment, 138
   retention, 138
   training
     bereavement syllabus, 165
     program syllabus, 197

W

Withdrawal of life-sustaining care, 139–140